VETERINARY VENTURES

Veterinary Ventures

by

R. Earnshaw, MRCVS

Memorable events in the life of a veterinary surgeon from college days in Dublin to retirement in Vancouver, British Columbia.

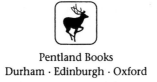

Pentland Books
Durham · Edinburgh · Oxford

© R. Earnshaw 2001

First published in 2001 by
Pentland Books
1 Hutton Close
South Church
Bishop Auckland
Durham

British Library Cataloguing in Publication Data.
A catalogue record for this book is available
from the British Library.

ISBN 1 85821 891 8

Typeset by George Wishart & Associates, Whitley Bay.
Printed and bound by Antony Rowe Ltd., Chippenham.

Contents

Contents

Illustrations

My gratitude goes to the late John van Zonneveld who encouraged me to write and guided me in the early endeavours.

Preface

While starting off in this endeavour I should perhaps offer a word or two of explanation. I am not a writer beyond an irate letter to the council or Prime Minister or in praise when Jack Nicklaus scored a hole in one. I have had a very interesting life and enjoyed most of it. The place descriptions are unreliable where memory has faded and I have altered certain people's names to save them embarrassment. The veterinary stories are for the most part as they happened, bearing in mind my recollection of many goes back fifty years.

Times change. My profession tends to model itself increasingly on the medical profession, the multiplicity of expensive tests having replaced the skills of the clinician. Operating room procedures backed up by ultrasound, sophisticated X-ray techniques, blood analysis and transfusion facilities which now compare favourably with the human medical counterpart are found in many veterinary hospitals.

Veterinary nurses now undergo two or more years of rigorous training and naturally expect remuneration commensurate with their experience. But it all costs money. Fees have escalated to offset these requirements which most of the public can afford. Many owners, however, can not meet the costs of spaying, neutering or vaccinating their pets. As a result unwanted offspring have become a sad problem.

If I have offended anyone with these writings I apologise. If I have embellished certain happenings I plead writer's privilege. If any readers have recollection of these events I would be very happy to hear from them. Write c/o the publisher.

My long time friend and financial consultant David Gowman has sent me a calendar every Christmas for the past twenty-five years. Accompanying each is a verse or quotation. The one entitled 'Success' appeals to me because it embodies my own philosophy. I read it often.

Success

Success is speaking words of praise,
In cheering other people's ways,
In doing just the best you can,
With every task and every plan,
It's silence when your words would hurt,
Politeness when your neighbour's curt,
It's loyalty when duty calls,
It's courage when disaster falls,
It's patience when the hours are long,
It's found in laughter and in song,
It's in the silent time of prayer,
In happiness and in despair,
In all of life and nothing less,
We find the thing we call success.

Anonymous

CHAPTER 1

The Beginning

My father, William Victor Earnshaw, qualified as a veterinary surgeon at the Ballsbridge College, Dublin, in 1924. After a few temporary assistantships he joined the British Colonial Service in Africa and was posted to Kano in Northern Nigeria. During his first tour of eighteen months my mother stayed at home to look after my brother, Desmond, and me, he aged two years and I six months. After my father's six-month leave my mother went out to Africa with him while we were parked with our grandparents in Ireland.

There was a succession of home leaves after which, at ages five and seven, we were sent to boarding school at Shepperton near London. The next tour of duty saw us with a distant aunt near Southampton. Whilst there we received the sad news that Father had died from a tropical disease. My mother would be returning to the UK soon.

It was a difficult time. Fortunately Mother received a small pension which enabled us to get by comfortably. Because of incompatibility in our natures one of the brothers was sent to boarding school while the other stayed home. We alternated.

My own interest in veterinary medicine began when I read some of my father's textbooks which were stored in our bookcase. Although I was still only fourteen years old, Mother encouraged me and began making plans for me to go to Ireland and live with an aunt while attending the veterinary college, some five miles away. First I had to pass an entrance examination. An equivalent one was that to Cambridge University, which I scraped through in July, a month before my sixteenth birthday. I was accepted as a first year student at the Veterinary College of Ireland. Classes would start on 15 September 1939.

The war with Germany was soon to commence. Call-up for military service was not until age twenty so I would be nearly through the five-year course before being conscripted.

Off I went by train to Holyhead then mail boat across the Irish Sea to Dun Laoghaire which was always a rough crossing. I looked forward to the experience although I had little knowledge of the animal world.

My aunt and young family welcomed me as a boarder but owing to the clamouring of three young children I felt my presence would be temporary.

Like other students enrolled at the Veterinary College of Ireland in Ballsbridge, Dublin, I attended classes in chemistry, physics, botany and biology at the National University in Merrion Square. On my first day at the university I, along with about sixty other youths, crowded into the Clare Room and sat in tiered rows of desks. Around 10:00 a.m. a mature, tall and stately gentleman entered the room and mounted the podium. He addressed us, 'Good morning, gentlemen – and ladies.' He spoke with a pleasant Irish brogue. 'I am Professor Mahoney. I will teach you the rudiments of biology. You have entered an honourable profession of which you will be justifiably proud. Some of you will reach great heights in your career. Some of you will become involved in humanitarian work in outlying places of the world. Some of you will make discoveries that will advance the cause of human life throughout the years. Let me tell you now about the Hippocratic Oath which will govern many of your activities.'

A brave individual in the front row put up his hand. 'Excuse me, professor, we are veterinary students, not medical.'

Mahoney went red in the face. 'For Christ's sake, why didn't you tell me sooner,' he blurted out. 'Well, it's a different story. You're going to face five years of study then enter a profession with little financial reward. Many of you will slosh around in mud and slurry on grubby farms where you'll be slow to get paid for your services. The local quack will malign you to his cronies in every pub. You'll be accused of having book learning but little practical knowledge. While you have the chance, take my advice and use the door.'

There was, as it is called, a pregnant silence. Then Mahoney smiled as no one headed out. 'The earthworm is perhaps the greatest contributor to the survival of the human race.' He regaled us with this priceless information as many of the more studious in the class scribbled this gem in their notebooks.

And so it went. Professor Mahoney did teach us biology with a humour of his own. 'In many species the anatomy is such that one testicle is positioned higher than the other. I can't' – he put his hand

2

deep into his trouser pocket – 'Yes, it's the left one.' Then, 'In the South Sea island of Irano the disposition of the sexes is such that males outnumber females five to one.' After a brief pause, 'Even some of our female veterinary students might stand a chance.' This was too much for Miss Donnelly who gathered up her notebooks and headed for the door, only to be further offended with, 'Don't rush, miss, the next boat doesn't leave until Saturday.'

It wasn't a particularly stimulating year academically but my new found companions and I more than made up for it as we took on the great city of Dublin.

Incidentally, Maureen Donnelly overcame her annoyance and returned to further regular classes in good humour.

CHAPTER 2

Student Dances

My short stay at Blackrock ended when I rented a nice room in Pembroke Park, half a mile from the College. The house was managed by two elderly spinsters who provided breakfast and an evening meal plus laundry service for two pounds a week. My fellow renters were a professional engineer, a cub newspaper reporter, and Tom, a medical student in his fourth year with only one more to go – theoretically. He had attended the College of Surgeons sporadically for the past twelve years in order to take full advantage of a legacy that paid handsomely so long as he was a student. I heard from a friend years later that Tom had yet to graduate. His main classroom was Neary's pub, just off Grafton Street.

The evening meal was the scene of many erudite discussions on the war, history, complex engineering projects and amusing personal experiences. My allowance of sixteen pounds a month allowed for a few extras. Mother paid the college fees including textbooks, and regularly mailed socks and other knitted wear.

There were no written college rules, though it was believed that suspension would follow upon any student being arrested. This did happen when two impecunious individuals started a fire with newspapers in the outdoor toilet of a pub in Ballsbridge. When the bar staff hurried off to fight the fire, the students helped themselves to bottles of whiskey then made a hasty departure. Unfortunately, they boasted of the exploit to the wrong ears.

Most teaching institutions had behavioural rules that also specified approved 'digs' or lodgings. One non-approved place in Baggot Street was notorious for hell-raisers. It housed about forty students, all male, often five or six to a bedroom. No girl in her right mind would have dared to share such company.

The dances put on by the college students' union were a shock. The first one I went to at the Shelbourne Hall was packed. Ten or more students milled around the front entrance where members of the dance committee tried to collect the two shillings entrance fee.

There followed a long passageway to the hall itself where a live band played all the latest tunes plus some Irish jigs. From the hall a stairway led to the gent's toilet, a spacious room, the floor of which was now the resting-place for four or five drunken young men. One of them had parted with his last meal and a few pints of porter. Students were climbing through an open window, having scuttled over the rooftops to find the 'free' entrance. At around 11:00 p.m. there was a surge of students into the hall when the money collectors decided they had had enough. There would be time for several dances and the chance of seeing a pretty girl home.

Vets' 'hops' were declared unacceptable by the management so we moved to Mills Hall in the same neighbourhood but that did not last long either. We booked three or four dances at the larger Olympic Dance Hall where a well-known boxer, Eddie Downey, was the doorman and chucker-out. The last dance was definitely the worst owing to fighting instigated by groups of students, either medical or engineering. Ambulances attended to the injured long after the dance ended. We were informed that a bond of £10,000 had to be guaranteed before they would permit us to have the hall again. The roughhousing that seemed to accompany the vets' 'hops' was a great attraction, not only for students but also for many of the lovely young ladies of Dublin. The only other suitable venue was the Mansion House, a very spacious hall owned by the City, located next door to the residence of the Mayor. The rent was high but, as all our dances had been packed, we took the plunge.

In final year I was secretary to the dance committee and co-opted several members of the rugby team to join. Before one dance, Davy Clyde, a wild character who had bid 10,000 guineas for a filly at the prestigious Irish Bloodstock sales without a bean in his pocket, announced that he and his gang would crash the dance at precisely 9:00 p.m. First we had to contend with a call from the Garda in response to the Mayor's annoyance at the din coming from the hall. Then Davy led the charge through the double doors. Paddy Gallagher, our biggest and strongest committee member, floored him with one magnificent clout that bloodied his face and sent his followers fleeing to the gardens with our more belligerent members hot on their heels.

We carried Davy to the washroom and cleaned him up then sat him on a chair in the hall to be viewed in his drunken sorry state by the rest of the crowd.

When I went to the front to compliment Paddy, he said, 'Anyone else who tries it gets this' – and smashed his fist into the wall panelling. He wore bandages on his hand for the next four weeks.

CHAPTER 3

College – Second Year

The second year of the five-year course was spent at the Veterinary College in Ballsbridge, a collection of older buildings with an imposing gated entrance over which sat the Royal Coat of Arms – seemingly ignored by the various patriots who passed underneath and were anti-monarchists at heart. Each block of offices, lecture theatres, the forge and some loose-boxes faced on to a central grassed area. This was the operating site for horses after some straw had been thrown down to act as a cushion for the recumbent patient. The final year students would crowd round to watch the intricacies of modern surgery demonstrated by Professor J.J. O'Connor. This well-known veterinarian had gained notoriety by operating on a famous racehorse called Windsor Lad. The operation was for chronic infection in the frontal sinus and was more of a chisel and hammer job than a delicate surgical procedure. Professor Martin Byrne succeeded him in 1939. He was a first class surgeon and teacher, and had a good sense of humour.

We were always addressed as mister by the staff, some of whom would be waylaid as they departed with their pay packets on Friday afternoons to join the poker game in the common room which went on often through the night. We had lectures on Saturday morning and regularly saw the remaining players together with numerous empty Guinness bottles and sundry paper bags which had presumably brought in chips, i.e. French fries.

The latest movies were screened in the leading cinemas on Fridays. The matinees with reduced prices attracted many students. As there was a requirement of fifty per cent minimum attendance at any one course it was the practice to have another student answer the roll call before each lecture. On many occasions an attendance of some thirty students would give a positive response to all seventy names called out, prompting Professor Alfie O'Dea to dryly comment, 'It's nice to have a full class.'

In second year I switched to a larger boarding house in Anglesea

Road, about the same distance from the college, where some fifteen or more students both veterinary and medical were accommodated three or four beds to a room. It was much livelier and mixed me with like company. My special friend, Bob Gilmore, was from the North, the only son of Hugh D. Gilmore, a well-known veterinarian who practiced at Kircubbin in Co. Down. Bob was in his late twenties, with a BA degree from Queens University. He was full of devilment. We went out on the town together, and flirted with girls from the Swastica Laundry, which was located opposite the college, and engaged in various pranks. I have not touched on the antics of students, particularly veterinary ones, because it bothers me. I will always regret the many ways we embarrassed good people doing their job. On Saturday nights, returning to the digs around midnight, we played poker till seven a.m. when, as a group, we went to first mass at Donnybrook church. After an early breakfast it was off to a well-earned sleep. Study in such an environment was always difficult owing to noise and interruptions. For several weeks before exam time cramming was done after everyone was in bed with the help of one or two benzadrine tablets which warded off sleep. The next morning's lectures would then be missed or slept through.

Exams were held at the end of each college year, supervised by an accredited scrutineer to avoid cheating. Next followed an interview conducted by a panel selected by the Royal College of Veterinary Surgeons in London who would travel in turn to each of the five colleges in the UK.

Holidays were always welcome. Bob invited me to Kircubbin for Christmas. His father, Hugh, was an elderly vet, one of the old school. He wore a white starched shirt with winged collar and dark tie. Outdoors he sported a bowler hat. He must have been in his seventies at that time. He enjoyed regaling us with the many exploits of his long career.

Kircubbin was a small almost three street town on the north side of Strangford Lough where a pleasant little harbour sheltered a few fishing boats and dinghies. Two pubs, four or five shops and many small farms kept the economy static. Gilmore owned some land adjacent to his house where a building was used for a monthly cattle auction. More importantly there were also a number of gathering pens in which fatstock could be mustered then driven through a weighbridge where two Government graders, both veterinarians, assessed the beasts' quality to determine the amount of payment that would be forthcoming to the farmer. Gilmore received two pounds for every beast that went through.

It was Christmas Day, 5:00 a.m. and still dark when Bob and I arrived at the dock to meet his cousin Henry and his two sons, both in early manhood, and a large black lab. named Sport. We loaded Henry's boat with our 12-bore shotguns and gear and headed out into the Lough, the Seagull 7½ h.p. outboard motor chugging us along at about six knots. When we reached the island third up from the Lough entrance we pulled the boat up on the shore then threw seaweed over it. The island was about five acres in area and would be covered at high tide. At this time the tide was just turning from low as dawn was peeping through in the east. We spaced ourselves about fifty yards apart and lay down, each pulling seaweed over our bodies to act as camouflage. Have you guessed that this was a wild duck shoot? When the tide came up and began covering the lower islands ducks in their hundreds flew up to ours. The shooting was hectic and Sport was kept busy retrieving downed birds to Henry. I shot off a box of fifty cartridges in little less than an hour and the barrels of my gun were hot. I noticed the sea water seeping up. Just about then Henry called us back to the boat while Sport still worked on the many downed birds. We gathered up one hundred and fifteen in two hours. These, apart from our own needs, would fetch two shillings each in Belfast market a few days later. Depending on our bag we would sometimes go to another island further up the Lough or more often look for wounded birds in the area. On this day it was back to port, a couple of hot rums at Henry's, quite near the Quays, then a short stroll home to a turkey dinner. If I could grade the fabulous days I have enjoyed in my lifetime this one would be very high on the list.

CHAPTER 4

Seeing Practice

One of the requirements for students presenting themselves at the final examination was to produce a book of case histories which had been recorded during at least six months of seeing both town and country practice with an accredited veterinary surgeon. For this privilege one paid the tutor a fee of a few pounds a week where he was cheap enough to take it. A list of available practices was kept in the office, where the name of Gordon Keating in Portadown, Northern Ireland, was suggested to me. I was interviewed and felt to be suitable by his father, a very pleasant businessman in Dublin City. I was to learn that the many jobs allocated to a student more than compensated for the so-called training fee.

I had completed my second year and knew a little about medicines, anatomy, physiology, and not much else, as I headed by train to Northern Ireland. It was the spring break. There would be three weeks to glean some experience of country practice. The toilet on the train had a notice which read, 'Do not use the toilet while the train is standing in the station.' Underneath was scrawled, 'except at Portadown.' I wondered why.

A brief call at the practice after a mile walk from the station sent me to digs a few doors away which had been alerted to expect me. The landlady, Mrs Hamilton, was plumpish, probably in her sixties, and happy to greet me. The people I met in the North were always full of fun, witty, generous and great to be with. In fact, the digs were the best part of my holiday. Sam Hamilton was a baker working for a large company owned by the Davidsons, located near the Catholic part of the town. He was a confirmed Orangeman. Little should be said about the troubles in a narrative like this but I became very much aware of the seething bitterness which was partly religious and partly nationalistic that had simmered – and sometimes erupted – ever since the Battle of the Boyne in 1779.

The practice was mainly large animal. The office and outbuildings surrounded a big yard at the back of Keating's house. A laneway led past other back yards to a road. There was a garage for a small Ford car and a stable for a cob (horse) and trap (two-wheeled carriage). As petrol rationing was severe during wartime many not too distant calls were made in the trap. It was a scary means of transportation as you were quite high up in an open cockpit with no seatbelt. Rastus, for that was the pony's name, did not get much exercise so made the most of it when called upon. The homeward trips were often at a canter or gallop. Only mighty tugs on the reins would slow him down.

Keating was a well-built six-footer with a handsome face and a shock of red hair. He wore riding breeches and boots, a sports jacket, waistcoat and a tie blazoned with horses' heads pinned to his shirt with a small brass fox's head, the much-admired image of a country vet. During the whole time I knew him I never heard him laugh and rarely saw him smile. He was efficient, demanding of his employees – me and Jake, the yard man – and brash in his conversation. I never liked him.

CHAPTER 5

Dog Stripping

On my first trip to Portadown, one day in late afternoon, all visits had been completed and I was about to return to the digs where the evening meal would be followed by something interesting. Keating asked me if I knew anything about stripping fox terriers. I admitted that I didn't. 'Well, by this time tomorrow night you will,' he said. At 9:00 a.m. the following morning he drove me to a house on the outskirts of town, gave me a penknife and told me Mrs Brown in Number 27 was expecting me. His parting words were a great help. 'I'll pick you up at one o'clock. Make sure you collect a pound from her.' The house was typical of the row housing in so many cities at that time: brick construction, very small front garden, two storey.

Mrs Brown proved to be a pleasant person. Her fox terrier named Alec was more amenable than many I had met previously. I put him up on the kitchen table, which had been covered with a blanket, and surveyed the mass of excess hair that covered him from head to tail. The technique is to grab some hair between your thumb and knife blade then pull hard, hoping to cut through the tough dog hair. First I had to ask if there was a photograph showing what he was supposed to look like. I was shown a picture of the all-Ireland champion of a few years back – a beautiful specimen – but it wasn't Alec. I felt hopeless and wondered if I should run for the door. But I started in and before long asked if there was a knife sharpener in the house. A whetstone and an oilcan were brought out. I was able to sharpen the main blade. The work was tedious but I plodded on. Mrs Brown brought a cup of tea and a biscuit, many of which were to follow in the next few hours. They helped keep Alec in a good mood. By 12:30 p.m. he was looking more like a fox terrier and I was beginning to feel proud of my creation. My fingers were sore and on the point of bleeding. Mrs Brown was delighted. Even Alec seemed to perk up as he seemed to appreciate his new image.

Keating's arrival was announced by a few hoots of the car horn. I collected the fee. An extra shilling was pushed into my hand. Mrs

Brown insisted on coming out to the car to address my boss. 'This young man has done a wonderful job, much better than the last one that came. I want to have him come every time.'

Driving back to the office I told Keating, 'I now know all I ever want to know about stripping fox terriers – don't ever send me out there again' – and he didn't.

Happily, the electric clipper has rendered such arduous work obsolete.

CHAPTER 6

On My Own

One Saturday morning Keating left for Belfast by train to attend a meeting of the Veterinary Association, which he did about once a month. He never seemed to enjoy or get much out of them. Upon returning he was usually ill tempered, referring to his colleagues as 'a clatter of bastards'. Before leaving he informed me, 'I'll be back at four o'clock. You can tell anyone who phones that I'm out on a case and will be busy till then.'

He wasn't gone more than fifteen minutes when a telephone call came from a farm near Lurgan which I had visited with Keating. 'It's Kevin Masters,' said an anxious voice. 'We've got a cow with the brain fever. She calved yesterday and has been staggering in the yard for some time. Now she's down and looks like dying. Can Mr Keating come out at once?'

I told him I'd try to get hold of Keating but to prop the cow up as best they could. It was eleven o'clock and Masters' calls came about every half-hour telling me how much worse she was. They had wrapped a wet towel around her head following the advice of a local octogenarian but she looked as if she was getting worse. This was the usual type of call that described milk fever in those days – acute mineral deficiency as a result of the blood calcium being transferred into the freshly produced milk. It didn't happen often since very few cows in that area were big milk producers. If not treated it could lead to coma and death after several hours. The lay treatment at that time was to pump air into the udder through each teat in turn, which was then circled tightly with some cloth strips to keep the air from escaping. The internal pressure would stop further production of milk. The procedure often led to infection and had pretty well been replaced by injecting a solution of calcium directly into the system, a treatment I had seen Keating give only once.

It was nearly 2:00 p.m. The latest call from Masters was desperate. I decided to try to do my best and hurriedly packed a bottle of calcium solution, some tubing with a flutter valve and suitable intravenous

14

needle into a bag. Off I went after leaving a note for Keating – 'Gone to Swanly Farm for milk fever.' I dashed into town and caught the Lurgan bus, which took me within a mile of Masters' place. It was still out in the country. I went into a nearby farm looking for some transportation but all that was available was a bicycle, the farmer having gone to market in the car. I pedalled furiously until a flat tire slowed me down. I threw the bike into the ditch and hurried to the farm on foot. It wasn't far to go now but had taken me the best part of an hour to get there. In the farmyard twenty or more people had gathered as word of the illness spread in the district. Other farmers came to give advice and relate stories of their own experience with brain fever. I pushed over to the cow and told them I was from Mr Keating's and was going to inject the cow. I did this very expertly, allowing the life-saving calcium to flow from the inverted bottle into the jugular vein of the now prostrate cow. Having completed the treatment I stood back to await results.

I became aware of a commotion in the crowd. Next, there was a cheer. Then Keating was at my side. He took stock of the empty calcium bottle and tubing. 'What the bloody hell do you think you're doing?' he shouted, as he started to pump up the udder with what looked like a bicycle pump. The calcium injection was beginning to work. The cow was returning to normal and tried to sit up, making it difficult for Keating to complete the pumping.

A cheer went up and someone shouted, 'It's a miracle that you got here in time, Mr Keating, pumping up is the only way.'

I retreated, threw the empty bottle and tubing into his car and retraced my steps to collect the bike and return it. Then I caught the bus back to Portadown. I didn't go in at all on Sunday. Let him feed and clean out the kennelled dogs. Let him wash his own bloody car and make up his own bloody medicines. My relationship with Keating was definitely deteriorating.

CHAPTER 7

Night Colic Case

It had been agreed that if there were a night call Keating would knock loudly on the digs' front door three times. I was expected to dress quickly then present myself in his yard ten minutes later. I usually made it.

On this occasion I met old Willie Savage, a not too prosperous farmer who was leaning against Keating's car. 'It's old Bess again, down with the colic, just like she did last April,' he told me. 'I rode me bike into town 'cos there's no bus and I'll get it tomorrow.' Yes, I thought and by the smell of your breath you had a few pints when you got here.

Keating stormed out of the house. 'Earnshaw, is everything we need for colic in the car?' he barked.

'Yes,' I replied, 'stomach tube, colic drenches, morphine injection, Epsom salts. What else do you need?' With no reply we piled into the small Ford 10 car, me squeezed in the back seat along with his other gear.

It was nearly 11:00 p.m. Our journey was to Bambridge, some seven miles away. It was mid December, cold but dry. A mile from town at the first crossroads a red light was waving back and forth. We stopped. I was aware of several uniformed young men with rifles, standing around. 'Where are ye going,' shouted the leader – 'Oh, it's you, Mr Keating. Well, on ye go then.' This was a unit of the B. Specials, a paramilitary organization which regularly patrolled the backways for so-called 'security reasons'.

Willie had been blathering continuously about one thing and another, then he asked Keating how much the visit would cost. 'It'll be two pounds ten for the night call then a pound an hour for as long as we have to stay,' Keating told him.

By now we were approaching the farm buildings down a long laneway. A light shone from a kitchen window. When the car stopped Willie jumped out, saying, 'Wait there while I get a lantern,' then made for the house. Fully five minutes later he returned with his lantern, opened the passenger door, thrust three pounds into Keating's hand and announced, 'The mare's better, you don't have to do anything, good night to ye' – and he was gone.

Curses, curses and more curses on the return journey. Finally Keating said, 'It's the second time I've been caught, but the first by Willie. He obviously found out that the trip home from the pub by taxi would have cost him five pounds. Let it be a lesson to you.' And I suppose it was, for in all my years of practice not one farmer has ever fooled me into giving him a ride home from the pub on the pretext of a colicky mare.

CHAPTER 8

Stirling

In the summer holidays, after my third year, I applied for a travel permit to visit Stirling in Scotland where my Mother was living. She had been bombed out of her home in Portsmouth with the loss of all furniture and household accoutrements. I travelled up through Northern Ireland, then went from Larne to Stranraer via the night steamer. I soon had a job on a farm within sight of the famous Stirling castle. It was general unskilled work at harvest time and I enjoyed it. I joined the local Home Guard and sported a smart khaki uniform with a small KOSB badge – King's Own Scottish Borderers. I travelled up to Redford Barracks in Edinburgh where I was interviewed by a Captain in the Scots Greys, a regiment still using horses then commanded by an Irishman, Colonel Hume-Dudgeon. I was advised that my knowledge of medicines would probably get me a position as pharmacist's assistant but if I were to stay on at college and qualify in two more years I could join as a Captain in the veterinary corps. Sound advice, which I was pleased to take.

While in Stirling I met some medical students who were filling in their vacation as helpers at the local hospital. I was more than happy to join the nightly poker game, which occupied the time between attending casualties and delivering babies. This introduction was to prove helpful at a later date. My previous military experiences at the OTC (Officers' Training Corps) at school proved an asset. I surprised myself by winning the rifle shooting competition held at the local armoury. My nine out of ten bull's eyes was not equalled during a two-hour wait in the sergeants' mess, during which time three or four pints of Youngers ale rendered me almost incapable of staggering up to the podium to accept the prize of some seven pounds. But I did so, gave an appropriate salute to the awarding officer, and mumbled that I would donate the prize money to the squad's comforts fund, which provided the beer when we had a social evening.

CHAPTER 9

The Mount Street Club

At the end of July, 4th-year exams were over. I was wondering how to spend the next couple of months when a notice appeared in the local paper. 'Required by the Mount Street Club, two university students to organize the social activities of the club's turf-digging venue near Rathangan, Co. Kildare.'

The so-called 'Club' was a registry for unemployed men who were willing to work for a pittance but at the same time get fed well and enjoy a healthy body building period of physical activity. I volunteered together with a medical student named Rutherford. We learned that there would be no pay but we would live as the men and receive a small allowance to provide suitable social activities for the fifty or so incumbents.

We were driven down to what proved to be large stables located one hundred yards from a stately mansion which was the residence of the Moore family. The stable buildings had been remodelled to provide a cookhouse, dormitories and a dining room to accommodate fifty or so people. It was strictly bare bones.

Rutherford and I had a separate room with spartan furniture and we stood in line for our food along with the men. By and large they were a cross section of indigents, some deserters from the British forces and some well-educated older characters who had fallen on hard times. We each carried a brown paper bag containing half a loaf of bread, a hunk of cheese and an apple when we trooped off to the bog to dig turf. The site was about half a mile from the stables on the perimeter of a huge area which was being harvested by machines scraping off the top layers of the turf. These were dried and compressed into briquettes which appeared more acceptable to the drawing room fireplace than the rough product, although they both produced a warm glowing non-crackling heat. At noon we had a break and lined up for a mug of tea brought out from the cookhouse. The toilet was – where you could find it – and sheets of the few old newspapers sufficed for you-know-what.

19

Rutherford and I were invited over to the big house for dinner. We proposed that a dancing board could be brought in on a Saturday evening and a local ceilidh band invited to play. All the villagers from the small town would be invited as guests. The Moores had been through this before and were more than willing to organize the evening for us and, more importantly, pay all expenses. On the due day, a Saturday, the boards came in several eight by twelve-foot sections, which were assembled between the two buildings on a reasonably level area of lawn. At 7:30 p.m. our band, a fiddler plus piano-accordion player, arrived and the dance began. Many villagers came by various means of transportation: horse, farm cart, tractor, bicycle, a few cars and much shank's pony. Our men watched the younger folk dancing as they gathered in groups of ten or twelve. I noticed bottles of Guinness being passed around. Some desultory singing came from the groups who also seemed to be closing in on the dance floor. A few of the men took partners and enjoyed the ceilidh music. At about 9:00 p.m., Ryan, a spokesman for the men, came to me, quite drunk, and pressed two pounds into my hand. 'I'm not feeling well,' he said. 'Would you go into town and get me a dozen Guinness.' It was about three miles across the bog on a gravel road to the nearest pub. I said I would then rode off on a borrowed bicycle. After buying the booze I raced back with head down and nearly collided with a rider going in the opposite direction. Our combined speed of some 20 m.p.h. would have made quite a mess if we had met head on.

Back at the dance some car headlights had been turned on in the gathering dusk. The noise was getting louder as the band blared out 'The Walls of Limerick'. To my dismay, a fight had broken out amongst a group of our chaps and some villagers. Ryan was glad to see me. After taking his half sack of bottles, he told me he would sort out the trouble. But it got worse. Women were screaming and now several wrestling matches between our own men were cluttering up the dance floor. The band had quit as most of the guests drifted away. Mr Moore came over from the big house to witness the scene of shambles now well lit by a harvest moon. 'Shall I send for the Garda?' he asked me.

'No way,' I replied. 'These fellows are having the time of their lives, working off a lot of steam and satisfying previously repressed grudges against their mates. I will stick around to make sure no damage is done to your place and guarantee everyone will be off to bed by midnight.' Needless to say, booze was at the bottom of it all. A supply of Guinness had been surreptitiously built up over the past couple of weeks.

Then next morning at least half of the men showed up at Sunday breakfast with bruises, swollen eyes and a few arm slings. Ryan stood up, swayed a bit, then made a speech. 'On behalf of all of us here I want to apologize to Mr Shaw and Mr Ford for our behaviour last night. They both worked hard to organize the dance which was paid for by the folks in the big house who I also want to thank. I've been coming down here every year for the past five. It was the best entertainment we've ever had.'

CHAPTER 10

The Clinic

During the final year at Ballsbridge students staffed the daily clinic for outpatients. Lame horses, dogs, cats and birds would be brought for treatment, mainly by those who could not afford the fees of a private veterinarian. We were supervised by the professor or lecturer of surgery. During short holidays only a few of us remained to conduct the clinic, which was a great opportunity to enhance our practical experience.

When a mature lady brought in her cat for a sedative before she took it in a proper cat basket by train to Cork, O'Farrell handled the case. He prepared a syringe containing a low dose of morphine, not remembering that while this drug is commonly used as a sedative in most breeds, it causes great excitement in felines. After the injection was given the seemingly satisfied owner departed for the railway station. Two weeks later she reappeared at the clinic and asked for the student who had helped her previously. She related the story of the cat within a crowded train compartment rocking the basket so violently that she opened it to take a look. The cat flew out, scampered over the other passengers then clawed its way up to the luggage rack where it sat glaring and spitting at the terrified passengers until finally settling down near the end of the journey. 'Young man,' she said, 'I want to tell you how grateful I am that you gave the sedative. I can't imagine what he would have been like without it.'

One old fellow came into the clinic and told me his herd of goats was not doing well. He wondered if it would be possible for me to come out and examine them at his place in Cabra which was on the other side of the city. I agreed to go on the following Sunday, but told him there would be a small charge for transportation. This prompted him to thrust a pound note into my hand. He wrote down a short description of the bus routes plus his address. When I arrived there, much to my surprise, Colonel Standish, for that proved to be his name, lived in a very nice house set back from the roadway in a well tended garden. The Colonel was one of the old school, attired now in a well cut tweed suit, neat shirt and what I presumed to be his regimental tie. He welcomed me warmly with a firm handshake and invited me into the house. After we sat down in his well furnished lounge an elderly housekeeper brought in a tray with cups of tea and a plate of biscuits, though it was only about two-thirty p.m. I was given a full history of the goat herd and scribbled some meaningless notes.

The Colonel employed a man to come in daily and do most of the management, including milking. The milk was supplied to the Mater Hospital where pediatricians believed it was more suitable nourishment for some of their patients. We moved out to the yard where I saw several neat buildings then behind them five or six acres of grassland on which about twenty goats were grazing. There was a nice looking Rover car in the yard. We went to the barn where Thomas, the herdsman, had tied up two fully-grown goats. I started to examine them, surprised that they were in poor condition in spite of what appeared to be excellent pasture and Tom's assurance that he gave extra concentrates. These were the first goats I had ever been close to and I couldn't recall anything in the textbook except that the billy or male goat had a characteristically unpleasant pungent smell which was very difficult to remove from one's clothing. My dilemma was solved when one of them had a bowel movement. I asked for a container to put some of it in so I could take it back to the college for analysis. Tom took care of this while the Colonel and I returned to the lounge where two glasses and a bottle of Scotch sat on a small table. Fully two hours later, after hearing about the wily Pathans of the Northwest Frontier and the determination of the Dutch farmers on the African plains commanded by General Smuts, I staggered out to find the bus stop. When inebriated but still ambulatory I found my way to a digs in Upper Mount Street where an attractive maid allowed me to sleep it off. I will always remember Sheila fondly.

The faecal samples were given to the parasitology lab which found a very heavy infestation of tricostrongyle eggs and larvae. In other words the ailing herd had worms. Using the second pound the Colonel had given me I went out there on the following Sunday and detailed to Tom the treatment to solve the problem. Each goat was to be given an appropriate dose of Phenothiazine. The medicine could be bought without prescription from any country supply store or veterinary chemist. A further description of the condition was briefly explained to the Colonel over three or four scotches followed by more stories of army life and battles on the Northwest Frontier.

Next a series of samples had to be collected each week to find if the treatments were effective. It became a pleasant way of spending a Sunday afternoon. I also realized that the Colonel was quite lonely and enjoyed our conversations as much as I enjoyed his Scotch. But there is a limit. After four or five weeks of parasite-free samples the goats were in much better condition. I bade the Colonel farewell, promising to return and check on the goat herd in six months time. I never did.

Finally the day we were all waiting for – the examination results were posted on the common room notice board. My name was amongst them, followed by the simple word 'Passed'. Those reading the word 'Failed' were not so happy. There were probably ten or more of them out of over forty who took the exam, some of them for the fourth or fifth time. A celebration (booze-up) was planned for the bar of the Theatre Royal at 8:00 p.m. Word was passed to our final year tutors who usually were happy to join us. Unfortunately, several of the failed candidates were wont to vent their spleen in a more than verbal manner on the professor whose subject had been their downfall.

Most of us had spent five years together, sharing both good and bad times. Several friends had dropped out of the course suffering from illness, principally tuberculosis. This was often latent but flared up, possibly due to the strains of student life and poor nutrition. I also suffered chest pains at the beginning of the final year. After several weeks of worry and convinced that the all too common TB had found another victim, I jumped on my bicycle and rode to the nearest hospital. It was generally understood that students did not pay for medical services so I explained my problem to the doctor and asked his advice. Should I leave my studies and seek treatment, which usually involved a long convalescence, or finish out the course? He sounded my chest then ordered an X-ray. One hour later as I waited in considerable anxiety he reappeared with a smile to tell me, 'You haven't got TB. You are suffering from a common condition in young people called pleurodynia or muscle pain.' He handed me a prescription which could be filled at the hospital pharmacy. Again a

24

long wait, after which I happily left the building, found my bike, and started off holding the large bottle of pink medicine in my hand as I navigated the busy traffic. On a sharp turn to the left the bottle slipped from my hand and went crashing into the gutter. I didn't stop but went on back to the digs quite happily. I never felt the pain again.

We had enjoyed sporting activities such as soccer, rugby and hurling, at which the 'vets' acquitted themselves very well. We had travelled together in groups to Galway, Cork and Belfast to compete against those universities. I had played soccer for the College team at all of these venues and regularly on a Saturday afternoon at a field in Donnybrook where the clubhouse was licensed to sell porter till all hours and which, after the game, reverberated to the lusty singing of traditional Irish songs. Although of an English public school background, I was accepted by all and I think I became in many ways more Irish than the Irish themselves. We shook hands, exchanged home addresses, and promised to keep in touch, little knowing what our new status in life would bring.

and went our respective ways, — — — (or some such statement)

CHAPTER 11

The Final Year

Throughout my training I had hopes of following in the footsteps of my late father.

As the end of the final year approached I never doubted passing the exams and wrote a letter to the Colonial Office in London to inquire about employment. The reply came after a few weeks with an extensive application form requesting a character reference from every school I ever attended. The forms were completed then sent off a few days after the examination results. Knowing it would take some time to receive a reply I considered seeking a job in Ireland while waiting.

I went into the college and talked to Professor O'Dea. He asked me if I would be interested in doing locums for vets hoping to take a summer vacation. I jumped at the chance and signed up for a couple. The first was at a small town in County Limerick called Rathkeale. The veterinary surgeon there, Sean Hutch, was getting married to the daughter of the local senator and planned to be on honeymoon for two weeks.

I took the bus from Dublin. The town was quite unique. The main street was concrete throughout. On Mondays it was the site of the weekly market when groups of ten or more beasts – cows, steers, sheep, pigs or goats – would be held in place by drovers with sticks while prospective buyers walked amongst them. Straw was thrown down at the store and hotel entrances and barricades were placed in front of shop windows. This was a relic of the past. None of the merchants could agree on the site of a new market which would tend to draw trade and business in that direction. When the market ended the street was hosed down and left spotless.

My accommodation was in a hotel on Main Street directly opposite the Donovan Pharmacy. The staff had been asked to take messages from farmers seeking my services and to supply whatever drugs or materials were needed. The Ford 10 practice car was also kept in their yard and left for my use. It was the first car I ever drove.

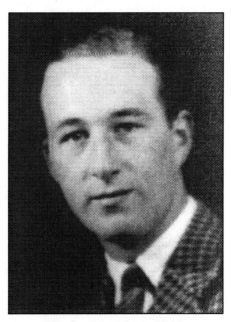

Final year student, 1944.

Sean and his new wife Mary popped in briefly to welcome me and impart a few suggestions. If there were major problems I was to contact Sean's father who was in practice in the neighbouring Co. Cork.

Dan Donovan was probably in his early fifties, a family man with two young sons. Always wearing a smile and ready to tell a joke he travelled with me for the first few days until I learned the lie of the land. The local farmers were pleasant and accepted me because I was helping Dr Hutch. After I had done two difficult calving cases and cured a horse with a bad colic I was accepted for myself. In a farming community the word soon spreads and can be the difference between friendship and hostility. Before long my departure from many farms was delayed by their hospitality, mostly in the form of half a tumbler of Irish whiskey. I found it necessary to take a siesta by the roadside on many afternoons.

Then came Listowell Race Week. This is was an annual affair similar to others held in different parts of the country. Many tinkers, gypsies, con men and sporting types would congregate for a week of festivities, and some horse racing. It was traditional that any household could sell whatever they wished during the week. Many tables were set up in front of their houses with bottles of Guinness for sale, possibly dusted off from the previous year, plus wee nips of something stronger. In addition, sandwiches and currant buns were offered. Dear old Dan felt that it shouldn't be missed.

On the evening of my second Monday we took ourselves, a couple of bags, and the train, over to the races. We found a sleeping room which was to be shared with four bookies, then headed out for a tour of the town, ending up at an all night dance which Dan left around 1:00 a.m. I had formed an attachment to a pleasant dancing partner and stayed on – and on. It was daylight when I crawled in beside Dan and, despite the grunts and snores of the other guests, soon dropped off to sleep.

In the afternoon we went out to the racecourse on the edge of town. Many tents had been set up by tipsters, three card trick men and fortune tellers. One chap had a bear on a chain doing tricks. All sorts of gear could be purchased, mostly stolen I would imagine. We telephoned the pharmacy. There were no serious calls. A few cleansing drenches and some mastitis powder had been dispensed and a lame horse was to be examined later in the week. We could stay another night. I sought out my dancing partner of the previous evening and further exhausted myself.

Dan had a pointer dog of which he was very proud. He asked me if I would like to go out one morning early to get some 'longtails', his terminology for pheasants. I jumped at the invitation. The two of us, accompanied by Chancey, walked the fields where there was good cover with our shotguns at the ready. The dog had an excellent 'nose' and could detect a bird twenty yards away. One cock was winged and fell out of range. Chancey followed the 'runner', as it is called, while we tried to catch up. At the top of the field he was crouched in an awkward position almost pointing. We searched all around him for the bird and finally, found it held fast under his paws. We had four cocks by 8:30 a.m. As the season hadn't opened yet we thought it wise to go home for breakfast.

I was invited to dinner at the Senator's pub, which was also his residence, and enjoyed a most convivial evening. This whole area had been the scene of many deplorable acts of savagery during the 'troubles' of the early twenties. First it was the British forces then later the civilian population which often pitted family against family according to their political allegiance. However, we didn't dwell on the past but played pontoon, which left me richer by a few pounds.

The sequel came fifty years later. Marilyn, my second wife, and I were touring Ireland by car, looking up the old haunts. Rathkealc was a much bigger place, as was Donovan's Pharmacy. We went in and stood aside while two middle-aged men waited on the many customers. Finally there was a breather. I went over and asked, 'Are you gentlemen Donovans?' Both nodded. I told them, 'Well, I knew your father a long time ago,' then related some of our amusing exploits to their delight. There were smiles all round. I was shown into a separate room in which Dan had preserved many ancient accoutrements of pharmaceutical interest, together with bottles of coloured fluids and noxious powders which had filled the pharmacy's shelves. I enquired after Dr Hutch and it was suggested that I phone his home which was on the outskirts of town. His wife Mary answered. When I identified myself we were both invited to come out for lunch. Sean was out doing meat inspection and would be back soon. Directions were simple and led us to a fine home in well-tended gardens. The greeting was warm as I told Sean I had come to return the fifteen pounds he had paid me in addition to taking care of the hotel bill. I said it was the best holiday I'd ever enjoyed. We sat down to a cold lunch with wine and reminisced about the old days. Yes, people had inquired after me for several years and hoped I would one day come back to take care of the practice.

Mary looked across the table at me. 'Ernie,' she said, 'do you ever remember me?'

'Yes I do, Mary, very well,' I replied, looking back at her. 'You were a raven-haired beauty.' My answer brought forth a little tear and a big smile – and then we were off to Limerick.

CHAPTER 12

Euthanasia – Putting to Sleep

This chapter is not for the faint-hearted. I am including it because veterinary surgeons are called upon to perform euthanasia for many reasons, often under difficult circumstances. The procedure may be hazardous and is always unpleasant.

The method used most often in dogs is to administer an overdose of anaesthetic intravenously. Before that technique was perfected we had a choice of the following:

Prussic or hydrocyanic acid administered by mouth. This substance causes paralysis of respiration and is the common content of the so-called suicide button secreted by spies somewhere on their person.

Strychnine by injection. This causes the contraction of all muscles including those of respiration, and thus stops the ability to breathe. Death by both these substances is caused by anoxia or lack of oxygen to the brain. Neither is painful.

Shooting with a captive bolt pistol or free bullet. This method is quick but messy and, depending on who is doing it, can be dangerous.

Electrocution – effective depending on the equipment which may at times malfunction. For this reason I do not recommend it.

During an early locum in the west of Ireland, I was called upon to put down a cow suffering from advanced tuberculosis. It was at a remote farm. Part of the exercise involved performing an autopsy then submitting portions of different tissue to the Government Laboratory. If the disease was confirmed in certain tissues, compensation could be claimed under an eradication scheme.

The poor beast was led by the farmer's two sons to a remote area beside a large river flowing towards the sea. I intended using a captive bolt pistol to stun the cow, thus rendering it unconscious, after which the throat would be cut to cause extensive bleeding and death – i.e. the system used in abattoirs. At least that was my intent. I discovered the pistol was faulty. I asked if there was a gun available but the answer was negative. I drove up to the farmhouse and picked up the only thing available – a large axe. To spare you the details I felled the animal with one mighty blow and carried on from there. When I had secured the necessary materials for the lab. I instructed the lads to dig a grave at least five feet deep and bury the carcass. The elder lad told me he would be going up to his first term at the Veterinary College in September. I said if he ever related the events which had occurred here, to remember my name was O'Brien.

A week later when I was in a different part of the country, I read in a weekly paper that the carcass of a disembowelled cow had been seen off the coast by an airline pilot flying into Shannon airport. His attention had been drawn to it by the congregation of hundreds of seagulls. It was rumoured to be the work of a certain cult. I suspected however that two farm lads had found it easier to dump the animal's remains in the drink rather than dig a grave.

CHAPTER 13

Castlebar

My next locum was at Castlebar in County Mayo. The west of Ireland is not noted for prosperous farms since the landscape is dotted with a myriad of rocks and stones, many of which have been gathered to build the noted stone walls thus clearing some pasture for the nondescript cattle and numerous sheep. The town itself was ancient, boasting one main street with shops on either side and three or four churches. The only vet in town was Dr O'Malley who picked me up at the railway station some distance from town in mid afternoon. As we drove the bog's narrow gravel road back to town in his weatherbeaten Ford 10 h.p. car he set out the rules of my employment. He would pay me seven pounds a week and also my hotel bill. I must not charge any drinks or extras. I must not spend any more time than necessary at his house where a nanny would be taking care of his two children while he and his wife went up to Dublin. Monies received must be entered in his daybook with a receipt given for all cash paid. Finally, 'This car is in excellent condition and I want to find it so when I get back.' He must have employed some young vet previously and knew what to look out for.

After being introduced to the hotel receptionist and leaving my case with her we drove up to his house which was in a prominent site on the main street, solidly built of grey granite, with attached garage but virtually no front yard. His lovely wife was already waiting on the doorstep with two suitcases. 'Hurry up, Pat, or we'll miss the train,' she called anxiously. With me cramped in the back seat amongst various overalls, veterinary instruments and other clutter, off we went to the railway station about four miles away. The instructions and many more were repeated: things I must do and must not do. Then they were gone and I now had to see what the car would do on the long straight narrow road back to town. With foot hard down I got her up to 40 m.p.h. when I saw the road ahead blocked by a herd of cows going home to be milked. My foot rapidly transferred from the gas pedal to the brake – but it didn't seem to make much difference. I blared on the horn and geared down into second but was still doing something like 10 m.p.h. when I was amongst them, still blaring the horn to gain a passage. It helped and I only bumped a few before I was in the clear. I didn't stop as the shouts from the irate cowman behind me became less discernable.

Back at his house the nanny, Bridie, made me tea. Two dogs came in for an examination, both with extensive loss of hair and scabby backs from continual scratching. The diagnosis was parasitic dermatitis which sounds very professional, but to the owners it was 'fleas'. Some appropriate shampoo was dispensed for the dogs and an erudite lecture on the lifecycle of these very common little insects which contribute so handsomely to the income of small animal practice.

It had been arranged that all messages from farmers would come to the house, usually by telephone. I would try to be there by 9:00 a.m. each morning. Bridie was a dear, probably in her early twenties, with a good figure, pleasant smile and happy disposition. She had been with the O'Malleys for two years and adored their two girls, one seven years old and the younger one four. I hung around until about 8:00 p.m. then went back to the hotel where I ordered a pint of porter to be put on my personal bill and a mixed grill to be ready in the dining room in fifteen minutes, allowing me to enjoy a hot bath. It was a good start. Over the next two weeks I did the farm work during the day, in many cases rectifying the awful mess some of the local quacks had inflicted on sick animals. There was also a religious connotation that was new to me when I saw crosses made of straw placed beside some sick beasts.

For the academics reading this the cases seen were known locally as felon, sturdy or gid, thrush, scab, staggers, fluke, foot rot, brain fever, heaves, worm in the tail, red water and TB. Most of the farmers were poor but kindly. The car was a menace. I called in to the vet's garage and explained the problem to the mechanic who told me brake shoes were on order which should be ready in a couple of weeks. Driving was hectic. Slowing down was a battle with the gear lever, especially going downhill. Fortunately there was very little road traffic at that time.

During the two weeks I castrated three colts – in the standing position – these having been brought into O'Malley's yard. In those

33

days the usual anaesthetic for this operation was the 'twitch' – but I don't want to describe it. I was never busy.

The mixed grills at the hotel replaced the usual beef stew. The pints of porter to wash it down were something to look forward to. But the happiest time was shared with Bridie in the evenings.

Finally, two weeks later, I picked the O'Malleys up at the railway station. The holiday had been a disaster principally due to the exorbitant cost of everything in the country's capital. I was due to get there again in little over an hour to catch my train back to Dublin. My suitcase was already at the house. On the trip back O'Malley swore the car wasn't handling well and hit the gatepost when he turned into his yard. Fortunately, it helped us stop. Inside his office I handed him £34 in cash and told him probably an equal amount had been charged on the books. He peeled off £14 then asked, 'How much is the hotel?' I said I would phone them. The bill was £11 for accommodation and £6 for extras. I had forgotten the mixed grills and whiskeys when I invited some friends in to play cards.

I said, 'It's only eleven pounds for you and six for me as I had some extra food and drinks, which I have already paid.'

He was pleasantly surprised as he had been quoted £20 for my accommodation. He hesitated a moment then asked, 'How much was your rail ticket?'

I told him, 'Three pounds for the return ticket.'

Again he hesitated, then said, 'I'm a damned fool but I can't let it be known that you worked out here for two weeks then went back to Dublin very little richer. Here is your bonus for all your trouble,' as he handed me twenty pounds. Then we rushed to the station where I barely caught my train. Very little was said on the drive out.

A few weeks later when I was in Scotland hoping to find a job I wrote to O'Malley and asked him for a reference, which might be a requirement for any prospective employer. It came by return. 'The police are looking for you. There are seven charges of dangerous driving. There are four charges relating to damaged property. I have been told you are a competent young veterinary surgeon, but you must not show your driving licence to any policeman in Ireland for a few years.' He did not know I never had one.

I did not send it to G.P. Male of Reading, whose advertisement for an assistant appeared in the *Veterinary Record*.

CHAPTER 14

Scotland

It was well into August. A letter arrived from the Colonial Office in London to inform me that a personal interview would be granted in furtherance of my job application. I gathered my few belongings, obtained a travel permit on the strength of their letter and went over to Stirling, Scotland. I stayed at my mother's house. I soon met up with some buddies at the local hospital with whom I had fraternized two years earlier. Before long they co-opted me as a member of the night time poker school. Surprisingly, their skills had not increased. I think the few I had played with before forgot I consistently overbid my cards but usually came out a winner. The games were interspersed with delivering babies, stitching wounds, plastering broken limbs and other emergencies to which I was invited as a spectator. Seeing human blood or witnessing injury usually nauseates me. My winnings at poker games ranged between three and five pounds on most nights, which would far outweigh a young vet's wages and led me to the bad habit of late to bed and late to rise.

To please my mother I picked up a current copy of the *Veterinary Record* from the local vet, then replied to several ads in the 'Situations Vacant' column. In talking to the local vet, I had cause to review my career ambitions. If I went abroad now I would tend to forget the rudiments of farm practice for which the college curriculum was designed. I could spend a couple of years in darkest Africa supervising the vaccination of a few thousand cattle but if I became disenchanted would find it difficult to get back into country practice at home. In the end it was the health of the country's livestock, an ever-increasing consideration, that determined my path of action. I accepted a job offer in Reading which came with the request that I travel there with all speed.

My mother was delighted. Her sacrifices over many years in providing both my living and educational expenses were finally showing promise of reward. She told me that Reading was a nice town. She would buy a house there and take care of me. Rotten bugger that I was, I thoughtlessly told her that I would prefer to live in digs as my style of living would not be compatible with her views on many things. A few minutes later I found her in the kitchen shedding a tear.

And so I entered the next phase of a full and exciting life – one that in later years would conjure up many memories of vibrant and happy times.

CHAPTER 15

Reading

I arrived at Reading Railway Station in the late morning of a dull, drizzly, October day. The journey from Edinburgh had been long and tedious. Hundreds of matelots and tommys all carrying full kit, mostly intoxicated, crowded every compartment, passageway and toilet. At each stop there was a rush to the station café in the hope of finding something more stimulating than 'railway tea', but mostly in vain. Getting the troops back on the train was a lengthy business. I believe several were left behind.

I knew little of Reading other than it had a large biscuit factory and a jail that had once held John Bradford who coined a phrase which always appealed to me. His remark was, as he watched some poor wretch being dragged off to the gallows, 'There, but for the grace of God, go I.'

And there went I dragging my ancient but sturdy suitcase through the heavy wooden gates of G.P. Male's Veterinary Infirmary on Friar Street. The office was on the right and a small animal clinic on the left. Folks clutching cats or dragging dogs were either trying to get in or trying to get out and created a busy scene. Inside the office I met a well dressed, handsome, middle-aged man who stepped forward with right arm extended. 'You must be Earnshaw,' he said as we shook hands. 'We've been expecting you. I am Norman Male. It's lunch time so why don't we take you to your digs then have something to eat.'

On the drive through town I was informed that the practice had been started in 1912, and now had three partners and six assistants. As the new boy I would do mainly small animal calls during the day and farm calls after normal hours. For the night calls I was to be provided with a car, and sometimes I would travel with a colleague. I had every second Sunday off, and my salary was the handsome sum of seven guineas a week. Old G.P. Male, known as 'the Governor,' still lived in the past and priced many of his accounts in guineas, which at one time were gold coins worth one pound and one shilling.

We arrived at a stately house on Eldon Road where I was

introduced to Mrs Burden, a friendly, middle-aged lady who was to mother me for the next four years. Next we went to a British restaurant and ate shepherd's pie followed by rice pudding washed down with weak tea. Norman emphasized the importance of exuding confidence at all times. If problems were to arise, which would be inevitable, there were several colleagues who would come to my aid.

Back at the yard we went into the office where I met Brenton, the junior clerk whose age was about fifty, and also Hubbard, a plump seventy-year-old who sported what looked like a morning suit with a stiff white winged collar and black tie. I learned to love both in the course of time, and enjoyed the antiquity emanating from them. We looked down the list of cases that had to be seen that day. Norman said, 'Here's one you could take care of but I hate to give you this as your first case. It's a constipated dog just off the Shinfield Road so it won't be hard to find.' I wrote down the address, looked at the map and made a few drawings of the streets leading there.

Next, Norman took me over to the small animal clinic and introduced me to Miss Fussel, who was the vet in charge of that department, and also Neville, another ancient who assisted her, unqualified, though very knowledgeable in the ailments of his feline and canine patients. Fussel said the dog would probably have to come in for an enema so I should just go and pick it up. Norman took me further down the yard to my transportation, a 12 h.p. Austin saloon car, bigger and better than the heaps I had driven in Ireland, all of which were falling apart.

Off I went, being very careful to drive slowly and get the feel of the car and its braking capabilities. Fifteen minutes later I turned into Carey Crescent and pulled up in front of No. 26. It was an ordinary semi-detached house with a small garden and lawn in front, all very neat. The front door was answered by a portly lady who gave me a pleasant smile. 'Oh, you must be Mr Male, come to take care of Toby,' she said of the fat, oversized fox terrier which was baring teeth and growling up at me. Mrs Newman told me poor Toby hadn't gone to the bathroom for nearly a week, since Uncle Harry had given him some pork bones which he really enjoyed. I could see this was a case for the clinic and I asked Mrs Newman to secure a leash on Toby and put him into the back seat of the car. I closed the back door on the end of the leash so Toby couldn't get at me; a wise move since the growls got louder and louder as I headed back.

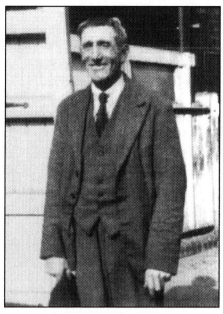

George, head groom, Male's Veterinary Infirmary, 1947.

When we arrived I drove down the yard then asked George, one of the grooms who was nearby, if he would get hold of the leash and take the dog up to Fussel. As George opened the car door, Toby hurled himself out and raced up the yard, his leash trailing behind him. Bill Thompson, another vet, was approaching so I yelled, 'Stop that bloody dog.' But it was no good. In less time than it takes to tell he was out of the gates, and by the time I got there all I saw was Toby, oblivious of the traffic, running at full speed down the middle of Friar Street. My heart sank. I would be fired. I would be sued. I would have to tell Mrs Newman I'd lost her dog. I went into the office to face Norman Male or even the Governor, but mercifully, only Brenton was present to receive the bad news.

He suggested that I telephone the police and ask them to keep a lookout for Toby, then slowly drive the same route back to his home. This I did without any sign of him until I turned into the Crescent. Toby was on his own front lawn and had made several substantial heaps, thus relieving his main problem. Confidently I rang the doorbell. A happy Mrs Newman was delighted to see Toby still performing.

'Oh, Mr Male, I'm so glad you could fix him up,' she said, 'And it didn't take a long time. I thought you might have to operate on him. How much do I owe you?'

I thought rapidly. Norman had not briefed me on current local charges. I blurted out, 'One pound, but that includes the transportation.' My first case at G.P. Male's had been a success.

CHAPTER 16

Digs and Dogs

The 'digs' were in a four-storey Georgian house fairly close to town and suited me very well. Mrs Burden, a handsome widow, had two daughters who helped run the place for six or seven boarders, all male. I was doubled up with Dick Early on the top floor. Dick was a Londoner with a job in a local office, living apart from his wife. He also played the clarinet, though better than I, and we often made noise together until banging on our door signified it was time to stop. Dick played with various dance bands at Saturday night hops in village halls around the countryside. He took me along several times, on the understanding that I would never be required to solo.

Also on the top floor were Harry Sloane, a newspaper reporter, and Tom Harris, a civil servant from Derby. Tom had recently been posted to the Department of Labour in Reading, and was an inveterate gambler, playing the horses by phone to a clandestine bookie during the day, then in the evening gambling at the dog racing track. After a few months he invited me along.

'How much would you like to win?' he asked.

'About twenty quid,' I replied – the equivalent of more than two weeks pay.

'Then how much would you be prepared to wager?'

'I'll bet ten,' I told him.

At the track we went to the betting area where the bookies were shouting the odds on the six dogs entered for the first race. 'I could put the whole ten down at two to one,' Tom advised, 'or more cautiously two pounds at five to one or anything in between.' We scrutinized the dogs as their attendants paraded them, and one in particular stood out. His name was Black Tom, and he was from Limerick, the breeding ground of many excellent dogs. The odds were two to one for a win. Should I gamble the lot? My ten pounds was more than a week's pay! I took the plunge.

Honest Joe Flanagan gave me the betting slip with the remark, 'The Irish fellow won't let you down, mister.' And he didn't, romping

41

home ahead of the others in great style. I collected my money then suggested a beer. Over our pints I scanned the race sheet for my next winner.

'You've finished betting,' Tom told me. 'You said how much you wanted to win and you've won it. Now is the time to quit. If you had lost your tenner that also would have been the time to quit. It's the main principle of people who make money at the track.'

I was impressed and happy with the evening's result but I never went dog racing again.

I soon learned that Reading was a pleasant town, which together with the suburb of Caversham straddled the River Thames as it wound its way towards London, some fifty miles further east. Picturesque villages and their bridges dotted the river every seven or eight miles. I recall the names Sonning, Pangbourne and Streatley, and more populated towns such as Henley. Each had attracted frequent visitors in pre-war years, and boasted many fine houses plus good hotels and restaurants, which were very scarce during the war.

Evidence of the war was everywhere. Public air raid shelters, uniformed military personnel, ration books for most commodities plus the nightly blackout were all routine. The continued bombing of Germany saw hundreds of bombers pass overhead each evening. A few doodlebugs landed in rural areas without doing any damage. We were spared the enemy rockets, which were aimed mainly at London.

Reading's London Road was usually packed with heavy transport vehicles bringing supplies from the western ports. Local government, a university, a large hospital, a cattle market and a biscuit factory ensured full employment in an area of prosperous farms, many of which were tenant holdings of large estates.

We usually completed the farm work by late afternoon. Often I would call in to one of my favourite farms for the evening meal, letting the office know where I could be reached in case of an emergency call. I was always well received and would spend the evening playing cards or going out to the local pub.

I joined the Home Guard at Peppard. We had a parade once a week for drill and target shooting at a local .22 range. After that it was the pub till closing time. We competed in athletics with other similar groups, and I recall being on the tug-of-war team which won against all competition. A number of us were asked to attend the local fete and bring along our running shoes. The organizers had persuaded a well-known sprinter who had won trophies to put on an exhibition 100-yard dash. On Saturday afternoon ten of us lined up in a field for the race. The star sprinter arrived decked out in shorts and shirt blazoned with insignia, and he also wore running spikes. When the starting gun went off we all surged forward to the cheers of the villagers. It was embarrassing when Harold Long, one of our mates, won the race in long pants and grubby running shoes.

CHAPTER 17

George Percy Male, MRCVS

The Governor was in his mid-sixties when I knew him. No more than five feet, five inches tall and of slight build, he had a kindly face and charming manner. He specialized in horse practice and was renowned throughout the country. His home was a pleasant Tudor-style house on the outskirts of town which he shared with his wife. They had a maid and a gardener named Musprat who also did odd jobs and chauffeured the Governor in his big American Buick. Musprat and the Governor made frequent trips to outlying stud farms and horse establishments, and I went along on many of these visits.

Of the assistants, I probably was the most physically able, and served as the Governor's assistant for the many operations he performed. Horses were brought to the Infirmary from distant places; there was stabling for up to eight. We performed the operations in a covered area well bedded with straw. The horses were cast using hobbles with the help of the two blacksmiths. I supervised the anaesthetic which was usually done with chloroform, and also assisted the Governor. My role included lifting feet, casting, floating teeth and supervising recovery. The Governor was expert at firing horses' legs which suffered from chronic sprains of the tendons, resulting in inflammation impairing their efficiency. The operation entailed drawing a very hot blunted blade across the skin over the tendons so as to burn in deep parallel lines half an inch apart, between the knee and the fetlock. The acute inflammation which this induced brought all the body's defences to the area and helped clear up the chronic condition. The procedure, called line firing, was done while the horse lay on its side under anaesthetic, and caused pain when the anaesthetic wore off and the horse got to its feet. For this reason we strapped a 'cradle' around the horse's neck to prevent him getting his head down and chewing the site. It was a barbarous procedure, yet highly effective in getting useless horses back to racing or hunting. I believe line firing is now prohibited by law.

Male had come to Reading at an early age to take over an existing practice. He hunted regularly and soon became known amongst the horsey set. A top dealer in the area named Oliver Dixon asked Male to vet a horse for soundness. Dixon hoped to sell his show jumper for a high price. For some reason the horse was unsound though would not appear so to anyone but an expert. When Dixon remonstrated with Male, insisting on a clean certificate, he refused, pointing out that Dixon would never trust him if he falsified a certificate. The men became good friends, and Dixon was a great supporter of the practice over many years.

One evening I telephoned the Governor about 9:00 p.m. for a case not far from his residence. It was for a pony with a very severe colic. I had been at the stable since 7:00 p.m. The grooms had given one of our #1 colic drinks as long ago as 4:00 p.m. when the trouble first started, followed by our #2 drench, both containing strong laxatives. But there was no bowel movement. The pony was in considerable pain and trying to lie down. I gave a warm soapy enema and had the pony walked slowly around the yard. The enema was expelled but nothing else. I passed a stomach tube and gave two quarts of warm water with epsom salts. Owing to the size factor I could not do a proper rectal examination. I was very concerned at the great pain being suffered and gave some morphine hypodermically soon after arriving. Unfortunately, it didn't seem to alleviate things very much.

I decided we were dealing with a twisted bowel which was untreatable at that time since it necessitated laparotomy or opening into the abdomen. I believe this has been carried out successfully at some teaching institutions more recently. The only thing to do was to end the suffering – but I wanted a second opinion. The Governor arrived looking very serious. After making his own examination and hearing the case history he agreed. I shot the pony and went home very depressed. Next morning at Tom Mays' knacker yard I did the autopsy and was able to display the twisted bowel to the two grooms who might have been sceptical of my diagnosis. The Governor complimented me for my action in calling him. Sir John Warwick, the pony's owner, was an old friend and long time client of the firm. He took the time to write me a short thank-you note from his parliamentary office. I still have it – somewhere.

I was to stay with the Veterinary Infirmary for four years, which were both challenging and enjoyable. I sometimes supplied the Male household with game, for which I was often invited to dinner on a Sunday evening. One time over the port and cheese the Governor told me that in 1910, Sir John McFadean, a senior professor at the veterinary college, had referred in class to a nuisance contaminant called penicillium notatum which was killing the cultures. It wasn't until 1928 that the Scottish doctor Sir Alexander Fleming realized the significance of this, and another twelve years passed before a team of Oxford scientists established penicillin's therapeutic use.

In looking back, I sometimes think my years in Reading were the best of all. Perhaps the following recollections will help explain why.

CHAPTER 18

An Early Case

One of my early cases in Reading was a greyhound belonging to a farmer at Peppard, about six miles north of Reading. Harold Long and his wife Jeanne became great friends, their farmhouse a second home during my four years in that area. Merrilass, their greyhound, had a great record, with several wins at the Reading track and a couple at Slough. Now she appeared weak, eyes and nose discharging, high temperature and off her food, the classic symptoms of distemper.

She was housed in a shed not far from the house, bedded on straw with pans beside her containing fresh water, cooked ground meat and sweet biscuits – all of which she ignored. Antibiotics had not yet hit the veterinary market, though from all newspaper accounts they were doing miracles with war injuries. I prescribed M&B 693, the most powerful sulpha drug available, and recommended that the discharges be cleaned up and antiseptic ointments applied. When Merrilass stopped eating and sank very low we began force feeding her with gruels plus a tonic to promote strength and appetite. I called in every other day for almost two weeks.

Finally there was a turn for the better. She ate some cooked rabbit and gained strength rapidly. A week later saw her out walking. But the worst was to come. The virus often damages the nervous system, manifesting as an uncontrollable 'tick' affecting any part of the muscular system or as paralysis of the hind-quarters. Merrilass developed the latter, and two weeks later I told Harold the case was hopeless. Norman Male came out at my request to offer a second opinion, which was in agreement with mine so Merrilass was put down.

My frequent visits to Peppard landed me all the farm calls in the surrounding area. I rapidly built a clientele of excellent farmers, many of whom became friends and enhanced my personal and recreational life. As a bright, handsome, young blade I was invited to attend many house parties, to shoot rabbits, fish waters, and join excursions to horse races and greyhound coursing. Unfortunately, having only every second Sunday off didn't allow for more than snatching a few hours when things were less hectic, which wasn't very often.

There were many calls to the office after 6:00 p.m., mostly of an urgent nature such as a difficult calving or prolapsed uterus or horse with colic or some kind of accident. We had a rota system where each assistant was on call first, second, third and so on. If the assistants had all been dispatched, one of the partners would fill in, but usually the first or second out was back to await the next phone call. Sometimes we would stop in at a pub to re-gather our strength – and wet our whistles.

CHAPTER 19

Small Animal Cases

As farm work kept me busy, house call visits to the Reading pets decreased. Male had wisely employed an older veterinarian called Atkinson to take care of them. When there were pets to be seen some distance from Reading, however, I would sometimes stretch a point and make a house call. One day when my brother was visiting we called at the Rothschild residence in Shiplake to check a Boston terrier's anal glands. These great little dogs are black and white and resemble bulldogs. They can also be quite feisty – and most certainly this one was. I placed him on the kitchen table and brother Des took hold of the collar while I began expressing the glands into some cotton batten. The dog growled, causing Desmond to jump back and release his hold on the collar. Next thing I knew, the terrier had my hand between its teeth and wouldn't let go for a painful five seconds that seemed like minutes. Bleeding profusely, I wrapped my wound with cotton batten and told Mrs Rothschild the dog badly needed treatment and should be brought to the clinic so it could be given a sedative before the glands were expressed. This was the only time in forty-five years of veterinary practice, thirty of which were spent entirely in small animal clinics, that I was bitten by a dog.

Then there was the poodle to be vaccinated against distemper at Caversham – this on my way back to Reading in the late afternoon. The owner answered the doorbell with a half-grown black poodle gripped in her arms. She said she had no means of getting to the clinic, and I soon discovered why. She was completely blind. We went into the front room where I prepared the injection. I gave her explicit instructions on how to hold the dog, which she said she understood. But when I plunged the needle into the neck area and the dog yelped, she threw up her hands, releasing the dog onto the floor where it fled under a couch. I looked at my syringe and saw the needle had broken off and was now presumably in the dog. After a lot of coaxing the owner managed to get hold of her dog and I felt around for the needle.

It was under the skin, so I told her that I'd have to take the dog to the clinic and remove the needle under local anaesthetic. It was nearly 6:00 p.m. Most of the staff had disappeared but head nurse Crowther was there and willing to help. I injected some local anaesthetic around the area, intending to make a small incision and retrieve what was left of the needle. I instructed Crowther not to poke around but to let the local take effect. I went to the office to make a brief phone call. When I came back I made a small incision over the site and searched for the needle – but couldn't find it. After poking around for fifteen minutes or so, I stitched the incision and said we would leave it for Fussel, the small animal surgeon, to take care of in the morning. Fussel repeated the procedure but had no better luck than me. The incision was sewn again and the dog taken home.

Fully a year later the Governor handed me a letter. It was from a lawyer's office claiming two hundred pounds for the loss of a poodle dog which had died as a result of negligence of one of Mr Male's assistants. Attached was an autopsy report from a neighbouring veterinary surgeon stating that in his opinion death was caused by the penetration of the left ventricle of the heart with what appeared to be a one and a quarter inch length of hypodermic needle, twenty-two gauge, but without its stub. Strange things happen. I think our malpractice insurance paid up.

CHAPTER 20

The Hopkinsons

O n a dreary, wet day in December I had finished the farm work as dusk settled in. There would be time to call at the office upon my return to Reading and do some booking before going to the digs for dinner. On Monday evening I was first call which almost certainly meant a trip to the countryside. It was 5:50 p.m. All but one of the office staff had departed when the phone rang. Brenton said there was a Commander Hopkinson on the line who wanted to speak to a veterinary surgeon. I took the phone.

'Can I help you, sir?' I said politely.

'Well, I hope so,' came the reply. 'I've just arrived back from the Med. on a few days leave and find that my wife has been hanging on to our old dog in the hope I could see her before she passes away. She has been very dear to both of us for many years but now is in a sorry state. I was hoping someone could come out this evening and put her to sleep.'

I asked the Commander where he was located and was told Basset Manor in Checkendon, an area I knew vaguely. It was a dark night and there were no signposts or streetlights. Our wartime car headlights were partially covered to send a beam only twenty yards ahead. But after a few more directions from the Commander, off into the night I went. Half an hour later I arrived at the church, just past which the Commander said he would be waiting with a flashlight to guide me into his driveway. Sure enough, there he was. He got into the car and we proceeded to his large country house. Inside I was introduced to his wife Jo, and poor old Bliss who was an aged Border collie. She lay on a rug by the Aga cooker in the kitchen. Border collies are very intelligent and make great companions. They are the most common breed used in herding sheep.

'She's fifteen, Mr Male,' said Jo. 'We've had her since we were married.'

I corrected her on my name and produced a stethoscope. Bliss was indeed at the end of the road. Her heart was weak and muffled, she was very anaemic and there was also a generalized enlargement of the lymphatic glands. I agreed that euthanasia was the best thing to do, and said I could do it by intravenous injection and I would not need their help. However, they both wanted to be present, and while I administered the painless lethal dose, each placed a hand on the beloved collie.

I was directed to a small washroom off the front hall to wash my hands while Bliss was wrapped in a blanket. The Commander suggested I wait in the sitting room which also led off the hall where the log fire blazed in the open hearth. After a few minutes he came in and said, 'Jo will be here in a few minutes then we'll have a drink, what would you like?'

'I'll have what you're having,' I told him.

When he left the room I settled into the comfortable chair and took in the impressive furnishings and many old hunting pictures that hung on the walls. Shortly the Commander brought three half filled tumblers. 'I thought a double brandy would do us all good,' he said, as Jo returned red eyed.

They told me the story of Bliss to whom they were obviously very attached, then Jo left for a few minutes, returning with a plate of chicken sandwiches. Peter (we were now on a first name basis) had replenished the same measure of brandy. We talked of many things – the state of the country, the war situation in far off places, plus the glimmer of hope for the future. It was nearly midnight when I stood up to go, but not until I promised to join them for dinner at the Manor on the following Wednesday evening. I do not remember driving home that night.

I soon knew Peter and Jo very well because I took on the care of their remaining dog plus the Jersey cow milked twice a day by Jo. I had the pleasure of sharing many pleasant dinners at Basset Manor whenever Peter was on leave, for which I was able to supply a pheasant or two.

After the war Basset Manor was reclaimed by the family that owned it, having come together since being scattered far and wide for many years. The Hopkinsons moved into a travel trailer, or what was known as a caravan, parked at Uxmore Farm near Checkendon.

I had not seen either of them for some time when I received an invitation to spend the evening. Peter was out of the service and they were going to emigrate to Canada. They had purchased a Jeep equipped with two-way radio so that they could keep in touch, Peter exploring the country ahead and Jo driving the vehicle towing the trailer. Although comfortable, they were fed up with Britain's post-war austerity.

Jo had come from Newfoundland, and although she did not wish to live there, she still had a love for the wide-open country where one could buy a good steak and a bottle of whiskey without a ration book. There was a problem, however. The severe restriction on exporting money (at that time six hundred pounds per year each) would not give them much to live on. Neither really wanted to work, other than to buy a property and build a home.

I usually had a brilliant idea for most things. After a couple of whiskeys I said, 'You know, throughout the war no pedigree blood stock has gone out to North America. Why not buy up some small pedigree dogs and take them out as family pets, then sell them for a bundle when you get there.' Little did I know that this suggestion would change their lives.

Fully two months went by. One evening about 6:00 p.m. a call for me came to the office. I took the phone, but all I could hear was a crescendo of yapping dogs. When the barking stopped, Peter came on the line.

'Ernie, we are living at Staines until we leave for Canada at the end of the week. Can you come up and see us before we go?'

With plenty on my plate and with severe petrol rationing it wasn't a good idea to leave the practice area, but, well – they were old friends.

'Yes,' I said, 'I'll come up at 8:00 p.m. tomorrow night. Give me the directions.'

Staines was some forty miles from Reading. It was late spring, still light in the evenings. Their house was set back some way from the road, a modest place in spacious grounds. I parked the car, went up some steps and rang the doorbell. Again there was a crescendo of barking. When the door opened Peter was nearly bowled over by a torrent of dogs bursting out to welcome – or maybe attack – me. They were corgis, some of which have a dubious reputation – but these were friendly. Corgis are great little dogs, tan brown with some white markings and full of fun.

Peter was laughing. 'Ernie, this one's Inky; she's the Welsh champion bitch this year. We got her for one hundred pounds. This one's Tara, the Scottish champion for three years running. Brownie won at Crufts last year.'

And on it went as he related their origin and cost, most of which was in three figures. They had bought eleven of the top corgis in Britain, which would go as pets to the New World. They thanked me for the idea then we had a few drinks followed by a nice dinner. But the barking was getting to me, so after promises to keep in touch I escaped a little after 11:00.

Several years later when on a visit to Britain I called at Basset Manor where I had first met Peter and Jo. I met the present owners who were friendly and told me that the estate, which held so many memories for me, had been declared a Heritage Home by the National Trust. We walked over to one corner of the extensive gardens to view the pet burial site. There were three small gravestones. On one of them was engraved 'Bliss 1944'.

CHAPTER 21

Ivan Coleman, MRCVS

A large veterinary practice is challenging and exciting, and affords many opportunities for a young veterinarian to improve his practical knowledge. One of my teachers was Ivan Coleman who was a partner living in a spacious house at the practice centre on Friar Street. He was the son of a veterinary surgeon who had practiced in Swindon, where I was destined to go. Unfortunately, Ivan suffered from a chronic form of undulent fever. The comparative condition in cattle is called brucellosis, a bacterial infection that causes abortion of the calf at the fifth or sixth month of gestation. Both diseases are caused by the same bacteria. It is presumed that human infection results from contamination during the removal of an infected placenta. There is a blood test to gauge the amount of antibody in one's blood, called a titre. Mine was 1:1760, which is high, probably resulting from small amounts of infection which were enough to build up a resistance but not produce the symptoms of chronic headaches. Nowadays, wearing arm-length plastic gloves minimizes possible infection. In addition, programmes of vaccination have pretty well eliminated this disease from cattle herds.

If Ivan had an interesting case he would ask one of the assistants to go out with him. He often took me to assist in preparing an animal for surgery or administering an anaesthetic. His services were frequently sought in the area where I did many of the calls. He would suggest to the farmer that he would like to get a second opinion from Mr Earnshaw, a newcomer to the practice, who had all the latest knowledge about the specific condition. It was his way of introducing me to the client – and very flattering to me. The next call from that farm would ask for Coleman or Earnshaw – and before long, the request would be for me. Many veterinarians are very jealous of their clients and don't want anyone else sharing them. Coleman was just the opposite.

One cold, wintery afternoon we were returning in his spacious American Ford from a farm near Basingstoke where he had been asked to give a second opinion on an injured racehorse. For several miles we followed a farm truck which he recognized as belonging to Jim Miller, a popular farmer from Mortimer. When nearing that neighbourhood the truck turned into the parking area of a pub and we turned in beside it. Out stepped Jim and Ewart Dance, another local farmer. We all went into the pub where a fire blazed in an open hearth. Jim made the first call. 'Landlord, we'll have four double rums, please.' We sat around a table, thawing out and enjoying each other's news. Coleman called for a second round of doubles. Then it was my turn. By this time we were mellowed and embarking on jokes and dubious subjects. An hour had passed very pleasantly and it was really time to head home.

Ewart struggled to his feet. 'Landlord,' he stammered, 'could we have three double rums – and one single.'

I was quick to add another suggestion. 'Please, landlord, make it two doubles.' The realization that we all needed no more rums soon became apparent, especially to those still with more driving to do. We thanked our host and left, feeling better able to face the chill of a late December afternoon.

Many years later when in Canada I read in the *Veterinary Record* obituaries that Coleman had died. I wrote to his widow and told her of the high regard I had for this good man.

CHAPTER 22

Dog Attack

Dogs worrying sheep is a common occurrence in country areas. It often happens with some of the best-behaved breeds when two or more dogs get together and roam around the countryside and come across sheep that are not fully protected by a secure fence. A latent savagery may surface. However, this case was quite exceptional, and the only one I ever encountered.

One morning a call came in from John Green who farmed near Henley. He said one of his cows had been attacked and killed by a dog. He asked if I could go to the farm and meet a police constable there at about noon. I arrived at the farm and we walked across the field to where a cow lay dead. She was old and in poor condition. Around the hindquarters I noted several deep gouges. On the ground pools of congealed blood were attracting flies. John told me the cow was a barren or non-breeding one used to suckle a few calves in the yard every morning. When he went to fetch her, he had seen a large German shepherd dog worrying the cow which was already down. He chased it off, and found the cow breathing her last gasp. He phoned the police, who suggested a veterinary surgeon be called in. John knew the dog lived at a house about a quarter mile away. He was upset and wanted to claim for his loss and ensure there would be no recurrences.

The policeman and I went to the house and met its lady owner. I explained that her dog might have caused the death of an animal, therefore I wanted to do some tests. She admitted the dog went missing all night, and took us out to her back yard to see it. With her help I gave the dog an injection of an emetic and while this was acting, clipped several tufts of hair containing dried blood. A few minutes later the dog vomited congealed blood and a large amount of short brown hair. I told the owner and the constable that this would indicate the dog had attacked the cow and caused its death. The constable advised the owner to keep the dog confined to her premises until further notice.

Two months later I attended the magistrate's court in Henley and gave my evidence. The constable stated the blood-covered clippings I had taken from the dog had been confirmed as containing bovine blood, as had the vomited material.

Magistrate Goldsmith, however, didn't buy it. He said the dog could have licked up the blood and hair if it came across the cow already down. He also believed the wounds could have been inflicted by a person at an earlier hour, and found it very difficult to believe a dog would do this sort of thing. Case dismissed. All John Green got was two pounds for the carcass from Tom May, the knackerman.

CHAPTER 23

Trigo

Veterinary students came to the practice for the major part of the college holiday. Most were eager to learn, and they helped break up the monotony of long drives into the country. Some took notes all the time. Some posed questions about diagnosis or treatment and were referred back to the textbook. Some were sceptical of certain procedures and critical of others. These ended up going with someone else.

When working fifteen or more miles from the office a country pub was the handiest place to eat lunch. In those days, the best fare offered was usually beer, bread and cheese, and a pickled onion. Good company made the sojourn enjoyable. One such student was Ian Munroe, a well-informed, mature young man who had been invalided out of the Royal Air Force after a dogfight with a German Messerschmitt. He had suffered injuries which resulted in the loss of one eye and a walking impediment. This may have incapacitated his ability in the cockpit but he was still able to step smartly aside when a flying hoof came his way – except this one time.

We were on our way to a horse-training establishment in Buckinghamshire, to put down an aged racehorse called Trigo. He had a most illustrious past including a Derby win, and subsequently sired several notable thoroughbreds. When we arrived a groom led out an aging thoroughbred which I think was in the upper twenties, a venerable age for a racehorse. A deep and spacious grave had been dug over to one side. The head groom, an elderly man, bow-legged from many years in the saddle, was either surly or sad. Speaking in an almost hostile tone, he told us we were to amputate all four feet at the fetlock joint. Apparently these were to be preserved and mounted in silver, one going to the Jockey Club, one to the Natural History Museum, one to the jockey who had ridden him in the Derby, and one to the owner. I asked the groom to bring me a stable rubber, which is like a dishcloth, and a container of crushed oats.

'What do you want them for?' he said aggressively. 'Why don't you get on with it – trouble is with these young 'uns they take so long doing anything.'

When the two items were brought I asked the under groom to feed Trigo. I then tucked the stable rubber under the halter on both sides, thus covering his eyes. He was munching away contentedly. I returned to the car, picked up the Greener humane killer which fires a free bullet, walked smartly over to Trigo, placed the bell of the barrel in exactly the right position then struck the firing pin with a small mallet.

Trigo dropped like a stone beside the grave. I returned to the car and searched for my post mortem knife, delaying things while a convulsive spasm seized poor old Trigo. Several minutes passed then the body completely relaxed. I meticulously checked for cessation of breathing, heart beat and palpebral reflex, then pronounced the animal dead. I handed the post mortem knife to Ian and told him what was required. I would go up to the big house and have a word with the trainer.

Half an hour later I returned to find the grooms shoveling earth into the grave. Ian was over by the stables wrapping the hooves in sacking. He hobbled back to the car visibly in pain.

'What happened?' I said.

'Well,' he moaned, 'I was stupid enough to go to the hind legs and at the first cut from behind I got kicked very hard which sent me flying. I don't know if my leg is broken or not.' This was no laughing matter.

'Get in the car,' I said. As we were ready to drive away the head groom left his shovel and came over.

'I don't know your name, mister,' he said, 'but I want to tell you I have seen many horses put down but I have never seen it done so well as you did it.' And he added, 'It's also the first time I seen a man kicked by a dead horse.'

CHAPTER 24

Hampstead Farm

My favourite farm was Hampstead, reached off the Henley Road by a quarter mile driveway. It was on a rise, with a view across the Thames plain. On a clear day one could see Windsor Castle. Jack Maidment was a tenant farmer of the Phillimore estate, which leased out many of the farms in that area. The house was delightfully old, boasting a south-facing covered patio attached to the lounge, which opened to a gently sloping lawn and a large pond surrounded by flowered banks. During the day the domestic ducks frolicked there while wild mallards flew in and out frequently. The ducks, Indian Runners, were called into a shed at night for their main meal plus protection from Mr Fox. In return, they would leave behind twenty or more eggs for the pantry.

On the west side attached to the house was a large greenhouse abounding in colourful flowers which were brought in to adorn the living rooms. To the east was a large vegetable garden with a wiring over the berry section to keep the birds from sharing – or stealing – the bounty of fresh strawberries, raspberries and currants, to name only a few. An ancient wisteria crawled over most of the brick walls, and equally old red tiles covered the roofs. The front garden was bordered by a hedge which separated it from the driveway, farm buildings and cow yard. This probably helped minimize the wafting farm odours, though this aspect of the agricultural scene never bothered me.

Jack Maidment was one of three brothers, all farmers. His wife Carol was a good looking and exceptionally talented woman, as evidenced by her flower borders, greenhouse plantings, house decorating, horseback riding, party organizing, and cooking. She regularly planned trips to London shows and horse races. She also won regularly when we played pontoon, also known as blackjack, which was a household pastime before television invaded the quiet country scene.

Their only daughter, Jill, was about ten years old when I first visited the farm to treat a cow called Frivolous for a chronic lameness. It was summertime and Jill was home from boarding school – the regular upbringing for the middle classes. But she was nowhere to be seen. Carol explained that she was very shy about meeting people because of chronic eczema covering most of her scalp. She made regular visits to a London specialist who had been wrestling with the problem for over two years with little improvement.

Looking back, I am amazed at my brashness, but I unhesitatingly, and without seeing Jill, said, 'I've got some stuff in the car that will cure it.' Before I left I brought in a six-ounce bottle of Male's eczema lotion which was a watered-down solution of Liquor Picis Carb. I believe it is a coal tar derivative. 'Just put some of this on once a day,' I instructed – and from day one there was improvement. A month and three bottles of lotion later there was no sign of abnormality, plus a good growth of blonde hair. Sometimes you just get lucky.

There was also an attractive Land Girl living in the house. These were females who were organized as farm workers by the wartime Government. They were given a fixed wage and wore breeches and green sweaters.

A German prisoner of war, Hans, came daily from the camp near Henley. A large truck dropped off individual prisoners at several farms in the area around 8:00 a.m., then picked them up around 4:00 p.m. After the war, Hans elected to stay on at Hampstead where he lived as part of the family. He was a good, conscientious worker and later married an English girl. They settled in a smallholding in Sussex.

Carol Maidment's parties were legendary. I attended one New Year's celebration, a full evening dress affair, with my current girl friend. After a few drinks and a scrumptious 'Duck à l'Orange' dinner we played party games. One of the games was called Treasure Hunt. Teams of four set off by car to find a list of up to twenty items, such as a soldier's tunic button, a copy of yesterday's *Times*, a walnut, an item of woman's underclothing from a vicarage, a bird's egg, some warm milk from a cow, and so on. The rule was that you couldn't go to a house belonging to any of the guests. It was crazy, yet most teams returned within the two-hour limit with an almost completed list. Needless to say some players were in a sorry state. Tom

Maidment ripped his dress trousers when he climbed through a barbed wire fence hoping to reach a cow and get some milk in a cup.

After a rest and a hot drink or a whiskey, we played a team game in which people were paired off but not husbands and wives. The whole house became the playground after the lights were turned off. The winners were the couple last to be discovered by the searching pair who had a flashlight. The laughter and occasional screams added to the excitement, but not everyone was enthusiastic. Before long a deputation of females demanded that some other entertainment be provided. Once things calmed down we played a card game called Farmer's Glory, in groups of six. Then it was time for bacon and eggs before going off home to recoup or maybe milk the cows.

CHAPTER 25

Pigs and Bull

One of my enjoyable clients was retired Colonel Brundell Bruce of Hazely Heath. He had the typical image of a high-ranking officer – upright stance, aquiline nose above a well-trimmed white moustache. He lived fifteen miles south of Reading which was not my usual area, but I enjoyed cultivating clients who had nice farms, attractive wives or daughters, or good shooting, or were liberal with refreshment. The Colonel would always invite me into his study for a drink, at which time we discussed the work that I had done, the state of the country, and the military tactics of the war. He raised purebred Aberdeen Angus cattle which had produced several prize bulls. He also had a large herd of pigs.

One of his breeding sows died suddenly for no apparent reason. I was called in to do an autopsy. My elder brother was on holiday from the Edinburgh Veterinary College so the carving up was his job. He was in his second year, having returned from a stint in the army. I had a pretty good idea what we would find, but let him plough through the abdominal contents, liver, kidneys and on into the chest. The lungs were congested, particularly on the side on which she lay when she died.

'Well, I can't find anything that looks diseased,' he said. 'Maybe she had a heart attack.'

'That is an excellent conclusion,' I told him. 'If you now cut into the heart you will find a tumour-like lesion on the left auriculo-ventricular valve. The condition was caused by a previous attack of swine erysipelas from which she had recovered.'

He exposed the lesion to the Colonel and his herdsman who were very impressed. I recommended vaccination of all the pigs. We returned a week later with the vaccine. The staff caught the pigs while my brother filled the syringes and I did the injecting. There were one hundred and ten all told. We were getting through them in great style with only a dozen or so left when my brother said, 'That's the last dose.' We would have to segregate the remainder and come back a week later. Driving back to the office I tore a strip off him. He learned there's always enough – even if you have to cut the dose down a bit for each one.

I was called out to the same farm on a cold night in November to treat a bull that was reported to be badly bloated. I took with me the leather probang, which was a long firm tube that could be passed down to the stomach through a mouth gag. When I entered the loose box there were several locals present. I recognized Monger amongst them. He was the local quack. I had done some work for him previously.

There was a history of having fed the bull potatoes which, I imagined, had not been cut small enough so that some became lodged in the esophagus. The bull was bloated in the stomach, in great distress, breathing heavily, and grunting in pain. On palpating the lower neck area I thought I could feel the offending object. We placed a gag into the mouth, lubricated the probang with mineral oil, then cautiously pushed it down, dislodging the potato as it went. There was a rush of gas up the probang as the offending potato was displaced into the stomach. The nine or ten onlookers gave me a rousing handclap.

'I'll go in and tell the Colonel,' I said, as I packed up my things. As I headed out of the door I stepped on something hard in the straw. Kicking aside the straw, I saw a probang of the inferior gum elastic type, which gave me some thought. In the house the Colonel graciously handed me a half tumbler of Scotch. I told him, 'I think we've unblocked him, but I will instruct your herdsman to chop the spuds up a lot smaller.'

After putting all my gear back in the car I went to the loose box where a couple of men remained. The light was on and the herdsman was rubbing the bull's back. It was breathing very heavily, still very distressed. The probang on the ground had disappeared. I asked, 'What the hell went on here before I came?'

The herdsman replied. 'Well, we let Monger know the bull was bloated and he said he had cured several before, so he came over and passed that thing down while we held the bull. It went down just as far as yours but it didn't seem to help, even though he pushed several times.'

The awful realization that Monger had passed his probang into the bull's lungs was a terrible shock.

I went back into the house and told the Colonel what I suspected. I said we would treat the bull to minimize infection but, depending on the amount of damage done to the lung tissue, the outlook was grave. Before leaving I gave the bull a large injection of Prontosil, a liquid type of sulpha.

When I arrived at the office the next morning there was a message from the Colonel that the bull was in bad shape so he had asked Tom May, the knackerman, to come and shoot it and remove the carcass. Later in the day I told the Governor about the case as a matter of interest. He said he'd heard about Monger from another source.

A few weeks after the unfortunate case the Governor handed me a typed letter. 'Have a look at this, Ernie,' he said. It was an official letter from the Consolidated Livestock Insurance Company which read as follows:

Dear Mr Male:

It is our understanding that one of your veterinary assistants attended a bull belonging to Colonel Bruce on 10 November. A claim in the amount of ten thousand pounds, the amount of an insurance policy with our company, has been made as a result of its death. I would therefore appreciate a full report concerning the diagnosis, treatment and autopsy findings. Please describe the status of your assistant and indicate if a second opinion was sought before the animal was destroyed.

Yours truly,

William Ward (President)

I handed the letter back.

'I would suggest, Governor, that you reply stating that the assistant in question has taken up a posting in East Africa, and as far as you know left the country last week.'

I heard nothing further, but am sure the matter was settled amicably as I attended the farm again many times, and always enjoyed the hospitality and conversation of Colonel Brundell Bruce.

CHAPTER 26

A Sad Case

One of the principal scourges of the dog world is the virus causing canine distemper. Vaccination against this disease is now commonplace, with booster doses throughout life. I have alluded to the condition in the story of Merrilass. Another case was a dachshund, on the outskirts of Reading, which I attended as a house call.

The dog was ten months old, the loving pet of a retired couple living in a beautiful home with maidservant, outside gardener and Rolls-Royce automobile in the garage. I was asked to attend daily, which was a nuisance conflicting with my farm work; however it was fitted in. I cleaned up the eye discharges and checked that Daxy was being given his sulpha medication. A room had been specially set aside for his comfort. He never completely stopped eating, which is abnormal in this disease, due possibly to the offerings of calf's foot jelly, fried chicken livers and cream cheese, all of which kept up his strength. After two weeks of excellent nursing he showed improvement, wagged his tail, and wanted to go walkies.

I was delighted but painfully aware of the nervous system complications which were a common sequel to the clinical manifestations. Two weeks later when he was out on the lawn he had trouble walking. His hind legs seemed weak for a few days then collapsed under him.

Again I made daily visits and watched a gradual progression into complete paralysis of the hindquarters. We were giving arsenical tonics and weak strychnine medicines to stimulate the muscular and nervous systems, but all it did was perk up the dog's front end and appetite.

I told the owners the prognosis was extremely grave. There was a remote possibility of recovery after months of nursing, but the percentages were closely related to recovery from infantile paralysis in humans – not good.

The alternative was euthanasia. The distraught couple could not face such an outcome and requested a second opinion with a small animal practitioner, who shall remain nameless, in a neighbouring town. An appointment was made for a few days hence. I mailed a complete summary of the treatments to date.

At the unnamed clinic Daxy was carried in, wrapped in a warm blanket. In the presence of the owners and myself the examination began. It was very thorough, culminating with the doctor tapping Daxy beside his eye, causing him to blink. He rendered his opinion: 'I think the dear little dog has an acute calcium deficiency which, unfortunately, has progressed beyond all hope of recovery. I am going to recommend euthanasia.'

I was flabbergasted and annoyed. I should have said – 'You damned old fool, you don't know what you're talking about' – but instead said, 'I don't agree,' and walked out. I felt I should relate the story to the Governor who told me I had done all that could be done. He had heard of similar ridiculous stories about the same consultant.

The account was sent at the end of the month, which the clients refused to pay. The Governor telephoned them and pointed out that the daily attendance and proper treatments were more than one could reasonably expect. He said the outcome was unfortunately common where the animal had not been vaccinated. I think they paid the next bill.

When I discussed this case with a colleague he told me about an unqualified 'dog doctor' living near Brighton, who willingly took on these cases in dachshunds whether caused by post distemper paralysis or slipped lumbar discs. He had visited the place where he found rooms in a spacious house given over to numerous dogs dragging themselves over linoleum floors wearing diapers but all seemingly happy. Food and water were readily available. The incessant barking at least indicated healthy lungs. The 'doctor' reported that 60 per cent of the dogs regained full use of their limbs but it could take as long as six months. His fee was one hundred pounds a month, payable in advance.

The same 'doctor' was often consulted on other cases. A certain titled gentleman came to him with the story of his spaniel which had an ear infection that had failed to respond to lengthy treatments from the local veterinarian. A second opinion had been given by the surgical department of the Royal Veterinary College in Camden

Town. It stated the chronic ulcers in the ear canal would not heal unless a surgical operation was carried out to expose the length of the canal, thus allowing drainage of the discharges. This had been done and great improvement followed, but after some time the dog started shaking its head again. The Brighton 'doctor' inspected the ear canal with an otoscope and found a silk stitch which had inadvertently been missed when the sutures were removed following the operation. It was nothing more than this stitch that was now causing irritation. The 'doctor' removed it but the owner was not told. Instead, the dog would have to come back every week for 'special' treatments; and it did for several revisits. In fact all it really needed was time and a sprinkling of talcum powder!

But the reputation of the Brighton 'doctor' was greatly enhanced.

CHAPTER 27

Early Sunday Call

I was never at my best on Sunday morning and now heard the extension bell from the downstairs telephone creating hell at the ungodly hour of 6:15 a.m. While room-mate Dick Early pulled the blankets over his head, I stumbled out of bed and made my way down two flights to the hall table which held the culprit. 'Hello,' I growled.

'Coleman here,' said the familiar voice. 'You are first call this morning, Ernie. Major Dixon at Henley has a cow with milk fever.'

'Okay, I'll take care of it,' I stuttered after a couple of yawns. This was an emergency. When a cow calves, hormones prepare the udder or mammary gland to be ready for the offspring's first meal. At one time the milk would have been produced in moderate quantities, but the selective breeding of dairy stock for maximum production now made it possible for more than several gallons, rich in calcium, to be secreted. The effect of this was to drain the blood circulation of this essential element. The symptoms would start as lack of co-ordination, then progress to inability to stand, loss of consciousness, coma, and death if not treated.

The farmer usually finds the freshly calved cow lying out, semi-conscious, looking bad. Administration of a solution of calcium borogluconate intravenously corrects the imbalance and a return to normal takes but a few minutes.

Soon dressed, I hurried around to the pub yard where I often left the car overnight, opened the gates, revved up the trusty Vauxhall and was off full speed through the deserted streets of Reading. Major Dixon was a good friend, retired from a colourful career in the army. He now farmed fifty acres a mile or so from Henley on the Reading road. Everything about the place was spick and span, freshly painted and well maintained. I don't think he had much knowledge of agriculture but he employed a first class dairyman to keep him on the right track. His farm was the site for the annual Henley Agricultural Show. One day it would become a million-dollar site for residential development.

Speeding through the outskirts of the city, I became aware of a loud ringing noise, and looking into my rear view mirror saw that a police car was following. I knew the Henley Road like the back of my hand. The Dixon farm was some seven miles away on a twisty road but with virtually no traffic so early on a Sunday morning. I floored it. The Vaux shot forward, leaving the constables and their Rover well behind – for a few minutes, anyway.

Gaining on the corners but losing on the straight sections, their damned bell occasionally rang out but that didn't stop me. Careering into the farm driveway on two wheels, I pulled over to a loosebox with an open door. My calcium bottle and tubing in hand, I headed inside.

Major Dixon was trying to support the cow's head, and his herdsman had wisely placed a straw bale to help it sit up. She was in a bad way. I rapidly inserted my needle into the jugular vein then held up the inverted bottle so the life-saving calcium solution would travel into the system. It was then that two puffing uniformed policemen appeared at the door.

'Gentlemen,' I said, 'I want to thank you for the escort all the way from Reading. You can see this was a matter of life and death with no time for explanations.' The policemen disappeared.

The cow was recovering rapidly so after giving the herdsman instructions about limited milking and suchlike, I accompanied the Major into the farmhouse where Mrs Dixon, a lovely lady, provided toast and tea. Some fifteen minutes later I started for home, and to my surprise, when I turned out of the yard there were the two policemen standing by their car. The many charges that could be brought against me flashed through my mind when one of the constables stepped forward, hand raised. I stopped. In a level voice he said, 'Excuse me, sir, we've unfortunately burnt the clutch out of our car. Would it be possible for you to tow us back to Reading?'

I always love helping the police.

CHAPTER 28

The Sporting Life

I've always enjoyed shooting even though there were few opportunities during my younger years. In my first job there were many. Since the war was still on, shotgun shells were hard to come by. Most farmers received an allocation from the War Agricultural Committee, ostensibly to shoot vermin, and used all that came their way. Maurice Rand, my good friend at the firm, gave me a single shot .22 rifle with aperture sights. To this I added a silencer of my own design, using part of a bicycle pump barrel fitted inside with round washers then secured over the end of the barrel. The normal loud crack became a soft pffffft, which could not be heard more than ten yards away. It was the ideal poacher's gun.

The countryside abounded with pheasant, many being raised commercially for the hotel trade or for his lordship's table. No tenant farmer would dare shoot one on penalty of losing the farm. We were often called out when the farmer would start his day at 6:00 a.m. or earlier to treat a beast in trouble, maybe a milk fever or calving. Driving through the Oxfordshire countryside early in the morning, free of traffic, was always a pleasure. The 'long tails' were plentiful along the hedgerows or around the hayricks. They could be picked off easily from inside the car on the way to the case, then retrieved on the way back provided the coast was clear.

Rabbits were everywhere and many wheat fields in early spring were eaten down to the ground for seven or eight yards from the hedges. This loss to the farmers amounted to some thirty million pounds annually on a national basis. The farmers all thought myxomatosis, a virus introduced from Australia a few years later, would kill off the rabbits and make them that much richer. It didn't, but subsidies did.

On a warm evening one could find a quiet place where rabbits abounded, then with a view of one hundred yards on either side one could sit in cover and shoot eight or more within the hour. You remained hidden. At each shot all the rabbits would bolt for cover of

72

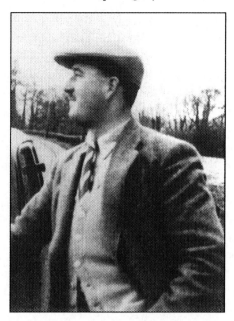

Country vet, Reading, 1947.

the hedge, hide for a few minutes, then venture out again. The country dwellers got most of theirs by setting snares or using ferrets to drive them out of their burrows – into strategically placed nets. If I shot more than I needed for the digs or friends I would gut them, then take them to the local pub for either the landlord or his customers, and was often rewarded with a pint.

We also shot rabbits in the wheat fields after the crop was cut and bound into sheaves. These were grouped together, ten or twelve stacked against each other, five or six yards apart in rows. If it was a fine night when we returned from the pub to Harold Long's farmhouse, usually about 10:15 p.m., we would take a shotgun and drive in his car down to the wheat field. The car had a sliding sun roof, allowing one of us to stand on the front seat with gun poised as the other drove around the sheaves with headlights full on. Rabbits bolted from the sheaves and became difficult but sporting targets. It took a good degree of skill as the car lurched its bumpy way. Time was taken retrieving the dead rabbits but in the space of twenty minutes we would have half a dozen. Then it was time to go. Someone would have telephoned Constable Wilson in Sonning Common to report the night shooting. He would soon be on his bicycle heading towards the sound of the shooting. We knew it would take him more than twenty minutes to get there.

As a local sportsman(?) or as attending veterinarian, I never learned which, I was invited to attend a deer shoot which was to take place on an estate near Henley at 11:00 a.m. on a certain Wednesday. It had been decided by the War Agricultural Committee that the deer in the park were consuming grass that could be sustaining cattle, which subsequently would help the war effort food supplies. A wooden stockade was built at the park entrance gate in the southwest corner. Beaters were to drive the deer from the park's hundred acres into the stockade, at which time the wooden gate would keep them in. They would then be shot by a gathering of some ten local sportsmen. After the slaughter a truck would be backed into the entrance to pick up the carcasses – or so it was hoped.

We brought along our twelve bore shotguns and were issued ten shells each, BB size shot. We lined up on the high side of the stockade, spaced about three yards apart, as the deer milled around inside. The committee chairman at the far end raised his gun and fired at the nearest buck. Before we could gather our wits some seventy deer surged towards the other end, knocking down the gate then fleeing into the laneway – and freedom. Several were dropped on the way. It became my job to see they were properly finished off. Ten unfortunate carcasses were taken to Henley to be dressed out. I think they ended up at Reading Hospital. Maybe this is the reason deer were always plentiful in the surrounding area. I wonder if they still are?

Pigeon shooting with a shotgun became popular as cartridges became more readily available after the war. I was lucky to get hold of several wooden decoys. On a bank holiday Monday, which also happened to be my birthday, I went out to Hampstead Farm where there was a field of ripened and badly lodged (beaten down by wind or rain) barley. I put several decoys out about thirty yards from a large oak tree while I sat well concealed beneath it. Before long wood pigeons flew in, some to perch in the tree for a few moments while others flew right in beside the decoys. I shot as they landed with wings outspread. They were allowed to lie where they fell as one mustn't be seen at all. I started the shoot at about 8:00 a.m., enjoyed a sandwich in the early afternoon then quit about 5:00 p.m. I picked up twenty-nine dead birds and carried them off in a gunney sack.

Back at the practice yard I washed all the flyblows from around their eyes and bloody areas. Next morning I sold them to a butcher in Henley for one shilling each. I had made more money enjoying myself than by working.

CHAPTER 29

Seamus Marshall, MRCVS

Since starting to write this treatise I have learned that my old – and best – friend has died. A letter from his wife, Kay, told me they were getting ready to go out. As he put on his jacket he collapsed then died almost at once. She later went through his many collected books, old magazines and, surprisingly, every letter I had ever sent to him. She enclosed one which, although it shows me up to be of dubious character, does reflect some of the aberrant thinking of youth at that time.

After qualifying, Jim, or Seamus as was his Irish name, did some government work in Northern Ireland. Next he came over to England to join a general practice in Salisbury, a pleasant city, famous for its beautiful cathedral. It was the centre of a prosperous farming area. On several weekends we visited back and forth. A year later he took an assistantship in Barnstable which is on the North Devon coast, an area of smaller farms with many narrow, twisty lanes to navigate. I made one trip down to see him after loading the car with three jerrycans of petrol from the practice pump. After a couple of years to gain some practical experience and make the many mistakes of a new graduate, especially learning to deal with overbearing matrons or skinflint farmers, he felt ready to start his own practice.

He selected a small town called Slane, north and inland from Dublin, where he put up his brass plate beside the front door. At that time this was the only means of letting the public know where your office was located. I visited him a couple of years later. We were sitting in his car when he made an exclamation.

'Got to go.' He had seen in his rearview mirror a corpulent matron dragging an equally corpulent, terrier type dog hurriedly up the hill – but it was too late. She caught on to the door, panting rapidly.

'When are you going to operate on Susan, doctor?' she asked.

'Well, now, Mrs Rafferty,' replied Seamus. 'She was only in season a month ago so she won't be again for five months. There's no great hurry – also just now my knife is away being sharpened.' It seemed to satisfy her. As we drove off, Jim said, 'That bitch is about five years old, has had several litters and, quite frankly, I'm frightened to tackle it. I think I'll send her down to the College in Ballsbridge to have the operation done there.'

He wasn't making money. After a few years he moved into the larger town of Drougheda where he prospered to the extent of buying one hundred and sixty acres of land just outside the city limits where he built a nice house. His dream was that the city limit would be extended to take in his parcel. He would then have a few hundred house building sites to sell. It never happened. Meanwhile he leased out the fields for grazing cattle and growing wheat.

Jim's family had grown to five boys and one girl. He was able to send them to good schools. Business was brisk so he could afford a locum, permitting him to take holidays. He and Kay came out to Vancouver for a visit. He was very impressed and berated me for not telling him what a wonderful place it was. But I am sure Ireland was his first love. After a couple of weeks, Kay returned to Ireland and work while Jim and I and a good friend, Jack Mellor, flew down to San Francisco where we stayed at the Fairmont Hotel. We saw Leo Gorschen perform miraculous imitations. We visited the Tenderloin one evening, which was an eye opener for Jim. Then it was on to Las Vegas with all its excitement. Jack and I flew home to Vancouver whilst Jim, after a few more days, took off for the Emerald Isle.

When Jim was in his late fifties he started to complain about Kay's cooking, which he said gave him indigestion. Kay was a nurse specializing in radiology. After weeks of listening to his complaints, she insisted that Jim go to see a medical doctor. An appointment was made for 2:00 p.m. the following day. In the morning he completed a tuberculin test on a herd of fifty or more cows and their offspring. By then his 'indigestion' was really bad. However, after a light lunch he presented himself at the doctor's office. It didn't take long. One glance from the medico and he called his nurse. 'Get a wheelchair here as soon as you can and phone the hospital that I will be admitting a patient immediately with a heart attack.'

Weeks of bed rest and medication plus an ultimatum to quit work or leave this world compelled Jim to sell his practice and live on Kay's income. He had bypass surgery then lived the quiet life, moving to Dublin where he hoped to be nearer medical expertise. He retained his local government appointment and travelled up to Drougheda once or twice a month to feel cows' udders for infection and also collect some rents. The Department was kind enough to let him continue this important though non-strenuous work.

Over the years I made two trips to Ireland when we would take off in his car and travel out to the west which he called the true Ireland. We enjoyed the pubs and meeting a few contemporaries who were getting fewer and fewer. In one parking lot he noticed a car whose inside was cluttered with veterinary gear. It belonged to a Dublin graduate, Tim Lynch, who had qualified before us. He had a big practice and told us he was doing well.

In later years my wife and I visited the Marshalls on trips to Ireland. Jim remained full of wit and good humour. He retained a unique Irish charm which endeared him to his many friends. His health was gradually failing so he needed to have further major surgery. We were visiting Europe a couple of years ago with a tight schedule of commitments. When I phoned Jim to tell him we wouldn't get over to Dublin on this trip he replied, 'Well, I will come over to London and meet you at the Regent Palace Hotel for dinner,' which he did. We had a happy evening talking over old times and he flew back to Dublin the next day. Kay told us in her letter that she was very much against him travelling because of his critical health but he insisted.

A true friend.

CHAPTER 30

Molasses

On a typical morning I drove to the practice about 8:30 a.m. and parked the car for Jennings to service while I scanned the office message sheet for the day's cases. After selecting a suitable number in a particular area, I transferred the names of the owner and farm to a day sheet on which the work done and medicines supplied were to be detailed. Once done, with a bit of chitchat, I assembled the required drugs and equipment and headed out with a mental note of the route to be taken and the urgency of each case.

During this routine our cars, all prewar vintage, would be gassed up, hosed down, and checked for the grind ahead. Veterinary farm practices were designated essential services to ensure livestock health. We had our own petrol pump with a generous allowance, which saved us the bother of dealing with commercial outlets and the required coupons.

We all drove too fast, careering down rutted country lanes without much regard for wear and tear. The average distance travelled by a country vet is about 16,000 miles each year. On many mornings we would go directly to a farm, perhaps to Tuberculin Test a herd, castrate a horse or vaccinate some pigs. I had arranged with the Fox Inn at Bix, near Henley, to provide a cooked lunch at 1:00 p.m. daily on weekdays. The Inn was very central to my general area, and allowed me time for a game of shove ha'penny with the locals and maybe a pint. The office knew to contact me there for further calls.

One day just before 2:00 p.m., a call came through asking me to go to the McAlpine farm at Fawley for an urgent case of milk fever. I was not the regular veterinary surgeon and therefore hadn't been there before. I thought their regular veterinary surgeon was from Twyford. When I drove into the farmyard a man rushed up to the car, obviously disturbed.

'You're too bloody late, she's dead,' he shouted at me.

I said, 'I'm sorry. I came twenty minutes after receiving the message.'

'Well we've been trying to get someone all morning,' he retorted.

'I'll take a look then,' I suggested.

The herdsman led me to a loosebox and inside was a very dead prize Ayrshire cow. Being freshly calved, she had a full udder and I noted that her mouth was sticky with molasses. 'What's your name?' I asked the herdsman.

'Leslie Ford,' he replied.

Pleasantly I said, 'Well, Leslie, tell me what happened here.'

'You can see for yourself,' he blurted. 'She had milk fever very bad and nobody was able to get here in time to save her.'

This statement was not reasonable as acute hypocalcaemia could be fatal – but not in a few hours.

'Do you want to tell me anything else, Les?' I prompted.

But all he would say was, 'You'd better go up to the big house and tell her ladyship.'

So off I went.

Lady McAlpine received me very graciously. I told her I was disappointed to have such an unfortunate happening on my first – and perhaps last – attendance at the farm. I said I wasn't satisfied as to the cause of the cow's death and would like to do an autopsy. The carcass would be removed to Tom Mays, the knacker, in Reading, after which I would report my findings as soon as possible.

Next morning I knew what I was looking for and so did Tom. The cow's lungs were full of the sticky water and molasses solution which Ford had dosed her with while she was in a half conscious state and not able to swallow properly.

That afternoon I called at the farm and related my findings to Ford. Poor Leslie sobbed as he admitted what he had done.

'Listen carefully,' I said. 'I am going to tell her ladyship that a mistake was made but that you in all honesty had done your best to help the cow. But if you ever lie to me again over a case it will cost you your job.'

Leslie appreciated how I handled the situation, and apparently so did Lady McAlpine for I became the farm's regular veterinarian. The new client was a great asset to the practice. Leslie and I became good friends.

more interesting chap. headings.

Bert and Bess

The war had almost ended with victory assured as the Allied forces closed in on the German capital. There were some farms that I rarely visited except to carry out routine Tuberculin Testing or clinical inspection of milking cows to ensure their good health on behalf of the Ministry of Agriculture. The latter would have been informed that our firm was the normal practice they would consult for veterinary services. But in a herd of some fifty dairy cows and young stock one would expect a few calving or stitching up calls, besides the supply of medicines. I hadn't been on the premises of Baltham Farm on the road to Hambleden from Henley for more than a year when there was a call to see a lame horse.

When I drove into the farmyard I was met by a German prisoner of war, who introduced himself as Herman and said he was in charge of the horses. At that time some one hundred and fifty German and Italian prisoners who were housed at a camp near Henley served as day labourers on neighbouring farms. Herman led out from the stables a huge Shire carthorse which stood seventeen hands high at the withers (just above the shoulders). A hand is four inches, so you can imagine the size of this beautiful specimen. He must have weighed a ton and was hobbling on three legs, with the off fore (right front), barely put to the ground. Upon examining Bert, as the horse was named, I felt excessive heat in the afflicted foot, and observed obvious pain when the hoof wall was tapped. I asked Herman to remove the horseshoe so I could search the foot very carefully. He fetched a set of shoeing tools from the stables, and without further talk lifted the leg between his knees and skillfully removed the shoe. Impressed, I remarked that this was obviously not the first time he had accomplished this task. He just smiled and nodded.

Then it was my turn. I pared down the sole until a blackened area appeared. As I cut further, pus spurted. Bert had apparently stepped on something sharp, such as a nail, which had penetrated the sole

with what

insert

into the soft tissues and set up a very painful infection. Herman was very pleased, and returned Bert to the stable where I gave him an injection of tetanus toxoid. I told Herman to bathe the foot then apply a bran poultice in a half gunney sack to keep the opening from drying out

? ?

My back muscles needed some rest before I continued on my rounds, so when Herman asked if I'd like to see Bert's younger sister, I readily agreed.

Bess was slightly smaller, in beautiful condition, with a glossy coat, hooves cleaned and varnished, and mane plaited in an attractive design.

I complimented Herman on his charges, and said I would call in a few days to see how Bert was progressing. A few weeks later I saw both horses pulling a plough on one of the farm's fields with Herman at the helm – a happy sight. Several months after that I visited the farm and was very impressed with Bert's and Bess's healthy appearance. Both were clearly 'show' specimens, so I asked Herman if he would be willing to exhibit the two horses at the Henley Agricultural Show, subject to the farm owner and camp commander agreeing. He quickly said yes.

Several weeks later Bert and Bess appeared at the show. They were led around the horse ring by two land girls who operated the milking parlour that Herman supervised, while Herman, accompanied by a soldier guard, looked on. The spectators applauded enthusiastically. As the veterinary surgeon to the show, I attended a free lunch in the Show Committee tent. During a pause in the President's congratulations to the organizers and exhibitors, I stood on my feet and said I had taken it upon myself, with approval of the show committee, to have the two Shire horses paraded, and wished to introduce the man who was responsible for their care. Herman entered accompanied by his uniformed soldier guard, took a dignified bow to the assembly, and was congratulated by the President. My announcement that he was a POW met with more applause, but I did not know his second name.

Eight months later the war was over. Things were returning to normal. We received a letter from the Ministry of Agriculture asking to have two Shire horses examined at Baltham Farm, Henley. A health certificate was to be issued to permit the owner of the horses, Graf Herman von Ziemen, to transport them to an address near

82

Cologne. I took the liberty of phoning the newly established European Consulate in London, and was told that von Ziemen had been the commanding officer of the 34th Panzer regiment. He had been captured at Benghazi and had now returned to his estate where he actively farmed over two thousand acres, including prize cattle. No wonder our veterinary services hadn't been required very often!

Our best client was Lord Hambleden, then serving with the army in the Middle East. His farms, Yewden and Greenlands, were attended frequently in response to the farm office's requirement that everything to support the cattle's health should be done. All calves were injected with B.Coli antiserum when born; milking cows were given mastitis vaccine; mineral supplements were made available to grazing stock; pregnancies were confirmed at three months.

The Yewden herdsman, Bloodwell, had moved twelve yearling heifers to a grazing field next to the church in the village of Hambleden. By some mischance a number of them had gained access to the cemetery part and were feeding on the yew trees whose leaves are very toxic to bovines. When the verger was notified he found help to chase them back into the field and latch the gate securely.

Word was sent to Bloodwell who telephoned Males who in turn located me at the Fox Inn, some six miles away. I called Bloodwell and told him that each heifer should be given a quart of strong ale as a drench after being confined to a small paddock in one corner of the field.

Fortunately there was plenty of help available. The local pub supplied twelve bottles of Breakspear's best. Not knowing which had eaten the 'forbidden fruit', each had to be dosed.

When I arrived the work was well in hand. Before long we had twelve yearlings staggering round the paddock ... inebriated, not by the yew, but by the strong ale. None showed other symptoms. After a while they were returned to the pasture.

Bloodwell asked if we would pay the publican for the 'antidote' ... and list it as medication.

CHAPTER 32

Extra Curricular Activities

At the beginning of the war most universities and colleges vacated London owing to the anticipated enemy bombing. It was a wise decision as many were demolished. The Royal Veterinary College moved to a large mansion at Holm Park, in the delightful village of Sonning. It was on the River Thames about five miles from the city of Reading. The first, second, and third year students resided at the mansion and were then bussed to Reading University for classes. The daily lunches there in the Buttery were also patronized by Male's unmarried assistants who found the fare and prices more attractive than those at the government-run 'British Restaurants'. The fourth and final year students were billeted in private homes at Streatley, also a delightful setting. The Bull Inn often reverberated on a Saturday night to the rendering of bawdy songs by the students, especially after a few pints.

Two of my lifelong friends, Harry and Tom, were at that time living in a caravan in the Sonning woods, having received permission from the Park Supervisor to camp within easy reach of the residence. They were third year students, given to the youthful debauchery of women and beer. They had their own brew barrel, which I replenished at Breakspear's Brewery whenever I could find the time. They also looked to me as the provider of eggs, vegetables, and the odd rabbit which I came across during my country rounds.

One evening I had been invited to a party at the National Institute for Research in Dairying at Shinfield. I knew several young people there who worked in an allied field, so I took along Harry and Tom as my guests. The sandwiches were abundant, fruit cake adequate – but the booze – wow! There were two rows of laboratory flasks lined up, one containing an orange coloured liquid which we took to be juice, and the other, a clear fluid which we learned via a whisper, to be absolute alcohol. The lab had anticipated a gathering of bodies such as us and had spent the previous month in providing the assurance for a lively evening. And it was.

The girls were very attractive, and we danced to recordings of 'In the Mood', 'American Patrol' and 'Elmer's Tune', at least while we could stand straight for the CHOH₂ was taking its toll. As the inhibitions of normalcy fast disappeared, we sought out the quiet of uninhabited offices with our more than willing female companions.

It must have been midnight when we left the place, our lasses clinging. And good Harry, ever the provider, had laden the back seat of the car with two flasks of orange juice and one of the clear stuff. Back at the caravan I was accorded the honour of being offered one of the single bunks which I was happy to share with my blonde companion who, for some unknown reason, changed her name from Rosie to Frances. With further fortifications of the NIRD cocktail, we sang a few bawdy songs, and gradually quieted down before passing out.

The next thing I knew, a female voice was saying, 'Ernie, wake up! We have to get to work! What time is it?' Sunlight streamed through the window. I bolted up and looked at my watch.

'Eight o'clock, hell, I've got to be at Henley by nine to castrate a horse!'

Frances chimed in, 'Let's get the hell out of here – bye Harry, and you, Tom.' Then I volunteered to take the girls to the nearest bus stop and we were gone.

So passed another social evening, and not so quiet night, in the annals of a young country veterinary surgeon.

CHAPTER 33

Bulls

I hate bulls. The many stories I heard as a veterinarian in large animal practice convinced me that there is a latent viciousness in all of them, similar to that in pit bull terriers. The depth of this belief caused me to have nightmares (usually after over-indulgence) in which I was being chased by an unusually large and vicious beast. I made my escape by waking up in a sweat.

Will Jones, who farmed near Henley, went out on a Saturday evening to feed his thought-to-be-docile shorthorn bull. When he entered the loosebox the three-year-old was standing quietly to one side and seemed to take no notice of him. But as he emptied a pan of concentrates into the manger, the beast struck him from behind so hard he fell to the ground. While the bull snorted and pawed the straw with his leg, preparing for a second charge, Will managed to wedge himself safely under the manger where he remained for two hours in severe pain.

The bull tried every manoeuvre to get at him, and eluded his attempts to grab its nose ring in an effort to gain some control. Finally, Will's wife, out of earshot in the farmhouse, came looking for him. She made several frantic telephone calls to nearby farmers and with difficulty they got a noose of stout rope around the bull's neck, attached the other end to a tractor, and pulled the beast, half choking, into the yard.

Will was taken to Reading Hospital where a fractured pelvis was diagnosed and treated over the next few weeks. The bull was taken to the slaughter-house the next morning. From then on the herdsmen were more than pleased to employ artificial insemination.

Another good friend of mine had a near tragic encounter with a bull through a little carelessness. Here's how it happened. Jack Maidment's Ayrshire bull approached him in the cowyard with snorts and head down menacingly. Jack aimed a kick at its nose but his other foot went from under him. He fell back onto the concrete and was knocked unconscious. Fortunately, Tom, the herdsman, looked out from the milking shed and saw the bull pushing Jack's limp body around the yard. He and another helper rushed out with pitchforks and prodded the bull back to its loosebox. Jack recovered rapidly and, after a hot bath, considered himself more than lucky.

Even the most docile bulls can be dangerous. An old Guernsey at Wargrave Manor Farm was treated as a pet by the aging herdsman in spite of my frequent and forceful admonitions. One day when he turned his back to exit the loosebox he was struck from behind and died from his injuries.

CHAPTER 34

Ready to Leave

I had been at Male's just over three and a half years. Not too many mistakes had been made. I was well received by most of the farmers and enjoyed a very active social life. At age twenty-four I was the senior assistant taking care of the clients in the more salubrious south Oxfordshire and south Buckinghamshire areas, perhaps including some of the best paying farm clients. I also drove the best car of the assistants, a 1939 Vauxhall 14, which was a bomb. My salary was the highest of the seven assistants. This was because I made an appointment to meet the Governor every six months and request a two pounds a week raise in salary. I was never refused – 'but don't tell the others.' This usually took place on a Sunday evening as we sat in his lounge enjoying port and cheese after a pheasant dinner. Male never offered a pay increase to his assistants. Fussel, the small animal assistant, was receiving only six guineas a week after working in the practice for six years. The girls helping with the kennel and grooming work came to the practice when they left school as sixteen-year-olds. There were usually twenty or more applying for this type of work. When they reached eighteen they would have to be registered with the Ministry of Labour and be entitled to unemployment benefits and larger salaries. Then they were let go.

The Governor talked a lot about interesting cases he was treating. One evening I broached the possibility of becoming a partner in the firm. He was, as ever, canny about discussing it but said he would talk with his partners: Norman Male, his son, and Ivan Coleman.

Nothing further was said about this but about that time a woman was employed as secretary in the office, one whose advances in my direction had been rebuffed. A feud developed. Other assistants were sent out to clients who had requested my services. Messages, some of them of a personal nature, were not passed on to me. She was not very nice. I spoke to the Governor about the situation but, as there was some family connection, he felt he could not interfere. My mind started to wander. Maybe it was time to move on.

There were a few small towns without a veterinary surgeon but I really wanted a country practice. After scouring maps and talking to many friends I decided to look at Wiltshire which was a county forty miles further west, an excellent farming area. One of my good friends, Godwin Pearse, said he knew one large farm there which would certainly employ me. On my Sunday off I borrowed a bike and took a train to Swindon, the largest town in the county with some seventy thousand inhabitants and the industrial centre for the Great Western Railway. About five miles further west was the small town of Wootton Bassett – in the heart of a farming district. I rode the bike out there, looked around and was impressed. There was a wide main street bordered by a few shops, a couple of pubs and terraced houses. An ancient town hall at one end was built on pillars. It dated back a hundred years to when the small town was a coaching stop for travellers on their way to Bristol, a thriving west coast port. There was a railway station and large factory for collection of the area's dairy products. Many of the town's four thousand inhabitants commuted daily to the busy factories in Swindon where there was also a four-person veterinary practice.

The blindness and ignorance of youth were my assets. My annual holiday was coming up in a few weeks and I told the Governor I would not be returning, thus giving him ample time to find a replacement. I wrote to a veterinary friend working in a distant and poor practice. The job was his for the taking if he applied right away. I told the Governor I would like to buy the many instruments I had become used to over the past years. He suggested I come to dinner upon my return from holidays and bring them with me.

A few weeks later I arrived at his home in my newly acquired Austin 10, circa 1935, which I had just persuaded a local dealer to let me have with a full tank of petrol for a fifty pound deposit. I lugged my large suitcase into his living room where we enjoyed a sherry together with Mrs Male, who expressed her concern that I was leaving. After a pleasant dinner we adjourned to his sitting room. Male said, 'Well, let's see what you have.' He was quite taken back when I produced a variety of syringes, forceps, shoeing tools, stomach tube, tooth rasps, castration knives, calving equipment plus various other useful things. 'Good Lord, Ernie, I didn't imagine you had such a lot of stuff,' he said, as we talked about the use and design of some of the instruments. The telephone started ringing out in the hall. 'Better put it all away, while I get the phone,' he suggested. He was gone for several minutes. When he returned I was sitting on the couch with my cheque book open and pen in hand.

'What shall I give you, Governor?' I said.

He hesitated for a few moments, wrestling with his thoughts, but finally said, 'You can have them all with our thanks for a job well done, but don't tell the others. We are sorry to lose you and hope you will keep in touch and come and see us when you are this way.'

Now I was embarrassed but managed to trot out, 'Governor, that's very generous – there's also the matter of a petrol allocation which has to be approved by you right away with the Ministry of Supplies.'

Sometimes I have qualms of conscience – but not often.

So I was moving on to another phase of my life. I was confident that I could build up a clientèle, do any farm work that came my way, and I would have the freedom to make decisions. It would have to be done on a shoestring.

CHAPTER 35

Setting Up

The great adventure began. One of my farm clients was old Mr Forrest, an octogenarian who had farmed in Wiltshire. He was a colourful character with a very broad dialect. He would come out with language such as, 'What be thee doin' then master.' Folklore dubbed such country dwellers 'moonrakers'. The name was based on the story of the villagers who hid their bottles of illegal alcohol in the village pond. When the revenue officers raided the village the locals, with long rakes in the pond, claimed they were raking the reflection of the moon out of the water. When I told him of my intention he claimed to be familiar with the area and volunteered to go there with me to 'show me the ropes'. But he didn't tell me he had left Wiltshire eighteen years previously.

We set off in my Austin through Newbury, over to Hungerford and up to Swindon. The main roads at that time had three lanes, one in each direction and one in the middle. We used to say the right side, the left side – and suicide. Only the brave or careless drove down the middle, sometimes flashing headlights in the hope that some silly bugger coming in the opposite direction would be chicken and pull over to his own side.

First of all we drove out to Wootton Bassett and had lunch in a local pub. I learned that old Mrs Spackman would occasionally take in a boarder and that a large room over the local undertaker's garage on the main street might be available to rent.

We inspected the undertaker's room first. The front door opened into a hallway that led to a small storage room. A stairway led up to a large room, which could easily be partitioned into two. It had a sink in one corner and several electric outlets. I made a quick decision to see the owner, Mr Wheeler, who agreed that my offer of one pound a week was acceptable. A short way further along the street I found Mrs Spackman, a delightful elderly lady who had a spare room. She was a widow with a thirty-five year old daughter living at home and working in a local drapery store. She would house me and feed me for two pounds a week. She agreed that I could have a telephone installed, which would be an extension from the office and could be switched from one to the other as desired.

I commissioned the local undertaker to produce a brass plate, thirteen inches by eight, with the simple words, 'R.E. Earnshaw, MRCVS, Veterinary Surgeon.' It would be mounted on a wooden backing and fixed to the wall outside the door to my office. My next visit was to the office of the local telephone company. At that time there was an exchange in the village through which all calls were passed by an operator. The company was very co-operative and agreed to the required installations. It would take two weeks.

The local newspaper ran a very modest announcement in two successive Saturday editions that a new veterinary practice would be starting in Wootton Bassett. It had to be carefully worded as our ethics committee frowned on anything suggesting advertising.

With a couple of weeks to organize, I ordered drugs, instruments and other equipment I would need. I went into town to buy furniture from Norman's, a second hand store, which was to influence my life considerably. The manager, Norman Wallis, treated me kindly. For a few pounds I acquired four chairs, a table and the desk he was using. The local plumber put in a gas-fired water heater while a carpenter partitioned the large room into a small waiting room and a larger one which would be my consulting room, pharmacy, and operating room and would hold the desk, telephone and typewriter.

Next came the job of finding a secretary to answer the phone while I would be out on farm calls. The 'Situations Vacant' column in the Swindon paper brought forth about twenty replies. On several evenings I called at houses and interviewed some bright, some dull, and a few suitable candidates for the job. My last, and successful, interview was with a pleasant young lady who had just left school and was an animal lover. She owned a spaniel dog. Although she lived in Swindon she would be prepared to travel out to Wootton Bassett daily to be there by 8:30 a.m. and stay until 5:30 p.m. She could pack a lunch and eat at Mrs Spackman's after switching the telephone. I was quite impressed and asked to meet her parents. How surprised I was when into the room came Norman Wallis, my friend from the furniture store. June Wallis became my capable receptionist. She never missed a day through inclement weather or illness during the three years she stayed with me. Five years later we were married in Canada.

The nearest 'opposition' was a 'quack' at Brinkworth a few miles away. I should not speak unkindly of the many unqualified animal doctors who acquired a degree of skill in their field, often by father to son teaching and experience – trial and error. They had no official recognition. Their methods were somewhat primitive since they had no access to modern drugs whose supply was restricted to either medical or veterinary doctors. But we kept our distance and our paths seldom crossed. More serious opposition was the firm of Hewer and Son in Swindon, a well-established practice with impressive premises and a few assistants. You will notice that I use the word 'opposition' which seems to be the universal term for one's veterinary neighbours. I believe the medics call theirs 'colleagues'.

My new digs were comfortable. Mrs Spackman provided a good cooked breakfast and evening dinner, which I was able to supplement with various fare from the farms. My room overlooked the main street and my car was parked around the corner. On the memorable day, 20 September 1948, the carpenter screwed the brass plate with its wooden backing onto the wall. I was ready to start my first veterinary practice.

CHAPTER 36

Opening Day

On the first day three owners with large dogs climbed the stairs to my office during the afternoon clinic, crowding my small waiting room. They each praised my coming, which saved them the long journey to Swindon. There were also some telephone calls from farmers wanting a visit on the following day. I felt these were going to be the bread and butter of the practice.

Within a few weeks my telephone was waking me up for early milk fever or calving cases which dragged me out before breakfast. It was very exciting to be my own boss – and depositing the cheques in my own bank account. Winter was approaching, a miserable time for the country practitioner as there were no heaters in the cars. Although veterinary surgeons were supposed to get some sort of priority in obtaining new cars, my number never came up.

As farm clients were established they were asked to notify the Ministry of Agriculture that Earnshaw was now their veterinary surgeon. From now on I would do the periodic mandatory regulatory work in the capacity of Local Veterinary Inspector. This included TB testing, brucellosis vaccination and udder checking for mastitis. It was routine work which could be done on my own timetable. It came in handy if things were slack. It also produced a sizeable cheque each month.

During winter it was dark by 4:30 p.m. but one still did farm visits. Cows might be in the milking parlour or cow shed as few were turned out into the fields, which were quagmires owing to the frequent rains. Dinner at my lodgings was followed by an evening of reading by the fireside. In time I made some wonderful client friends to socialize with. The telephone exchange was notified where I could be reached in event of an emergency.

The practice grew rapidly. Travelling further afield necessitated the purchase of a larger vehicle. It also enabled me to speed up to Reading for the annual Farmers' Ball when it was held.

Several small animal calls came from Swindon so it seemed

expedient to have a branch clinic there. In County Road I found suitable premises with a large garage at the bottom of the garden which I purchased after a treasured and loveable aunt provided a generous loan. Before long my evenings were spent seeing dogs or cats from 7:00 p.m. till all hours. My waiting room would be crowded and often there was a queue of people with their pets down the front path and sometimes along the sidewalk. This was a walk-in clinic. The two nurses working with me hurried the cases through. It was also a cash only business. Notices to this effect were prominently displayed in the waiting room. All surgical cases needing anaesthetic were scheduled for a Wednesday, which became hectic. The Swindon house calls were made either before or after the evening clinic, sometimes up to 10:00 p.m. Adding to this there often was a late farm call – maybe a cow with prolapsed uterus at Ashton Keynes – some fifteen miles away.

Letters came sporadically from my good friends the Hopkinsons who had settled in Canada at McDonald's Corners in Ontario. They had purchased eighty acres of woodland on the bend of a river about fifteen miles north of the city of Perth. They had built a house which included accommodation for the many dogs they still owned. Several of the latter had been entered in shows where their quality was recognized by winning prizes whenever they were in competition. Puppies had been born which were in great demand and sold for upwards of $200. The veterinary advice I had given by mail was appreciated to the extent that a letter arrived, forwarded from Reading. It suggested that if I were at all interested they would finance me to set up practice in Perth. It was a very generous offer but by this time I was tied up – or was it down – in my own practice in Wiltshire.

One day a telephone call came to the office while I was out doing farm calls. Mr and Mrs Hopkinson were having a party at the Curzon Hotel in Park Lane, London, that evening. They hoped I would join them. What a hope.

I mulled over the thought, realizing that it would mean a lot to talk over old times, good and bad, as we had done so often in the past. I decided to make every effort to get there.

All cases at the evening clinic received short time. I was able to get away by 8:20 p.m. I drove to the railway station and was lucky to catch a train at 8:40 p.m. Trains didn't travel very fast in those days.

It was an hour later that we struggled into Paddington station. A taxi ride to the Curzon brought me there just after 10:00 p.m. When I exited the elevator on the floor of their suite the boisterous sound of a happy crowd reached me as the partygoers spilled into the corridor.

I approached cautiously and entered the large crowded room. Peter and Jo saw me and hurried over. 'My gawd, you made it,' shouted Peter above the din. 'Jo, get your coat and let's get the hell out of here.'

We took a taxi to a fashionable restaurant where Peter ordered a bottle of Champagne and three lobster salads. They told me of their happy life in Canada and the many exploits with the dogs. They also reiterated the hope that I would take up their offer to go to Perth. This time the answer was 'maybe'.

These were sixteen-hour days. It was obvious that a second veterinarian was needed. In the summer of 1951 my elder brother graduated from the Royal (Dick) Veterinary College then came to work for me, moving with his wife and young son into the living accommodation at the Swindon Clinic. He was provided with a car and all necessary equipment.

The workload was eased, but the worry increased as irate farmers, quite justifiably, complained of his methods and lack of experience. By putting the best face on it and explaining that we both had a job to help him get into the routine, none left. In time they liked and respected him and were not upset when he became their regular consultant. But practice was not for him. After less than a year he applied for and took a teaching position in the Sudan and off he went with his young family.

The hectic pace of life had its effect on my health. Not through dissipation, but through irregular meals and worry, I developed chronic indigestion, which manifested itself in heartburn after nearly every meal and during the night. No ulcers were detected. I became Rennies (antacid) best customer. A half teaspoonful of bicarbonate of soda in a glass of water was equally effective in reducing the acidity when they were at hand. This condition has to a lesser degree followed me through the years. Fortunately, modern preparations to reduce gastric acid have come to the rescue and eliminated the discomfort and inconvenience of the past.

I was making a very good income specializing in infertility treatments. Some farms were twenty miles away to which I made regular visits and set up systems in which every cow had a case card on file. Records were meticulously kept. It was an innovation for many and proved itself to the extent that several farms before long had a surplus of calving heifers that were no longer required as replacements for infertile cows and could be sold. Several farmers asked me to spay their young heifers, which would fatten like steers and not come bulling. It was a great success. I replaced my brother with a series of assistants but for one reason or another none were kept for long. My receptionist, June Wallis, left to take a position in London and gain more practical experience.

The year was 1953. I took stock of my life. I was nearly thirty, overworked, unmarried with little time off, lots of responsibility and bags of worry. Believe me, the jollies exemplified by Siegfried Farnon are few and far between. I had travelled very little, just the odd jaunt to London. I decided it was time to sell up then go and see the world.

CHAPTER 37

Sunny Nutland

One of my early clients was a young man named Sunny Nutland. He lived with his aged parents at Lower Salthrop on a tenanted farm of some two hundred acres. He was the younger of two brothers, still unmarried at twenty-eight. He managed the farm, including a dairy of some fifty Holsteins, and regularly produced root and hay crops which were surplus to his own needs. He loved agriculture in all its aspects, supported the local hunt and encouraged his neighbours to avoid using barbed wire in their fences, and cut their hedges to make suitable jumps for the hunting horses. The hunt master, the Duke of Beaufort, often called to talk with him about local conditions.

When time permitted I was invited to shoot over his property, mainly rabbits and other vermin but occasionally snipe on a neighbouring farm's marshy area. He built a pond and stocked it with rainbow trout which grew to several pounds. I think these were to look at rather than to eat. We socialized together, often being the centre of boisterous activity at the young farmers' dances.

At the Harvest Ball we had a bowling (underhand) competition using the turnips which had been put on display, hurling them the full length of the dance floor during the interval. Another time we took the motor horn off an old truck then went to the cinema. We sat in the centre of the downstairs. At appropriate moments we sounded the horn, to the amusement of the patrons but consternation of the attendants, who patrolled the aisles hoping to catch us and throw us out – but we were not caught. One winter's evening we drove down to Bournemouth with two lovely young ladies to take them ice skating in the newly opened arena. It was a round trip of one hundred and twenty miles.

Sunny married and moved out of the farmhouse into one of the farm workers' cottages. It wasn't a happy union and ended in divorce a couple of years later. His second wife was to be very different. Mary had her own farm accounting business which contributed greatly to the record keeping of the farm. Sunny's parents passed away. The farmhouse was modernized where necessary and the happy couple settled in to raise a family of a boy and a girl.

Whenever we went back to England, which we tried to do about every fifth year, we stayed at the farm for a few days. Sunny took us on interesting trips such as Peter Scott's wildfowl sanctuary.

It was a great honour for me when in the late 1960s Sunny wrote that he would like to come out to Vancouver for a visit and bring his father-in-law. They stayed at a local hotel. During their first week I drove them to several farms where they spent the day with kindred souls to learn or at least see how we did things here. When I was able to take more time off we drove up to Princeton, far from the coast, to meet friends of my earlier days. The first visit was to Abe and Mona Willis who ranched over 6000 acres near Princeton. The drive up was delayed by heavy rain. It was 2:30 p.m. when we arrived for lunch. Norman, Sunny's father-in-law, was curious as to the identity of the delicious meat which he couldn't place. Abe told us it was from a mountain sheep ram he had shot in the Kootenay Hills. The prize head was being mounted by a taxidermist in Oliver which we were to see a few days later. After lunch Abe took them both in the pickup truck to view the Herefords grazing on the surrounding hills. They were intrigued when a coyote was spotted. Abe did his best to pick it off with his 30-30 rifle, which was always kept handy.

Over the next couple of days we called to see several old friends in the area where I had practised for nine years. We drove over to Percy Williams' spread in Beaverdell where we rode ranch horses – western saddle – over the hilly country.

Back at the coast we went up to Secret Cove where Don Pye took us salmon fishing. Norman hooked a big spring salmon which he played expertly following our advice not to rush things and let it tire itself out before we would use the net. It was reeled in up to the boat several times over the next twenty minutes. Then there was one last dash for freedom when it again plunged to the deep, so-called 'sounding'.

'I've lost it,' he moaned, as he reeled in slowly. He brought to the surface a large salmon head with at least four dogfish hanging on to three or four inches of its body. A sea lion had robbed us of our supper. However, later at the Jolly Roger Resort, the cook was able to save a couple of salmon steaks, which they both enjoyed.

Sunny left two prints by Harrison of woodcock in flight, which I had framed.

Some time later a letter from Mary told us that Sunny had developed a serious health problem for which there was little hope of cure. The following year, while in the UK, we went down to Swindon where we were met at the railway station by Sunny and Mary, then taken to the Goddard Arms Hotel for lunch. In the afternoon Sunny and I went trout fishing on the River Avon. We talked about the good old days. He had badly failed. After dinner back at the farm his nephew came over and took me rabbit shooting, then when it was nearly dark we went up to the pond to shoot wild ducks which regularly flew in from the town's parks. We bagged six in a quarter of an hour.

Time was running out for Sunny. His son was summoned home from Australia to take over the management of the farm. His daughter came home from her boarding school overseas. It was a sad time.

Sunny passed away quietly, leaving a legacy of many good friends, several in high social circles who valued his company and happy disposition. The Duke sent his personal condolences.

A couple of years ago Marilyn and I went down to Swindon, then took Mary out to dinner. We heard all the family news. She is living in a delightful house not far from the farm and was planning the garden landscaping. We still keep in touch.

CHAPTER 38

The Gilbeys

Wilbur and Margaret Gilbey lived in a large mansion at Cliffe Pypard, a parish bordering on the downs about seven miles from Wootton Bassett. For those who don't know, the downs are the extensive chain of hills located several miles from the south coast. Their main characteristic is a thin topsoil over chalk. Quite near was one of the so-called 'white horses'. In a bygone age the locals had removed the topsoil extensively, leaving the image of a horse some one hundred yards long and nearly as high which could be seen for miles. I never learned if the Gilbeys were related to the famous gin distillers. They were both in their forties. Their mansion, probably over one hundred years old, looked like a large cement block with little architectural merit. The grounds were immaculate and the horse stables in good repair, a credit to the staff.

The Gilbeys spent their days horse riding, going to horse races or shows and generally enjoying themselves. They hosted house parties for some twenty or more people to which I was often invited as a single. I had taken care of their two horses for minor ailments and treated two Labrador-type dogs. They were often in trouble, Jasper limping home one day with a broken leg and Meg suffering from poisoning which almost finished her.

The Gilbeys did not pay their veterinary bills. I had only been practising in the area for three months when they sought my services. In the three months that followed their bill mounted to over one hundred pounds. Accounts were sent out at the end of each month. If not paid at the end of the second month the bill, with its additions, would have a little add-on sticker sporting the word 'Please'. Next month in my handwriting, 'Would you please settle your account.' I was no longer invited to the house parties but had been invited into the house for a pre-lunch cocktail when I called to vaccinate the two dogs. Then one evening Wilbur telephoned to ask me if I would go over to Gloucester to vet a horse which he wished to buy as a birthday gift for Margaret. The visit would take most of a morning. I pointed out that the charge could be in excess of twenty pounds. I told him I would only go if he promised to pay his total bill, something over one hundred and fifty pounds. 'Good Lord,' he exclaimed. 'Margaret has been very forgetful for not taking care of it. I will certainly have a word with her.'

I drove fifty miles to vet the horse. It was at some large stables near the beautiful city of Cheltenham. The horse was a four-year-old grey gelding, about sixteen hands high, looking very fit. The routine was to check each leg in turn for any swellings or abnormality, then the teeth and eyes. Next I had the horse saddled for me to ride and test for wind. The groom held the bridle until I had my boots in the stirrups then let go. Without any prompting the grey took off like an express train, down the field at full gallop. I could see the far fence looming up rapidly and pulled firmly on the reins to slow him down. It didn't. I was faced with a collision, a jump of the four-foot fence or being thrown off when he finally came to a full stop. I remembered talking to Male about this situation and rapidly followed his advice by sawing the horse's head from side to side with forceful pulls on the reins. He slowed down and stopped a few yards from the fence. If I had had a riding crop I would have taught him a lesson there and then. As it was we trotted back to the stables where the groom and manager were waiting. When I dismounted I said, 'This horse is a bloody menace and will one day kill someone. It should not be offered for sale.' Then I left.

In the evening I telephoned Gilbey and told him the horse would not be suitable for Margaret as it had a tendency to bolt and was extremely difficult to control. 'Yes,' was his comment, 'We had been told that.'

My blood boiled. I lost control. I exploded. 'You devil, you might have warned me. I could have been killed by that damned horse. Mr Gilbey, I shall expect you to pay your bill at my office within one week. If you fail to do so you will hear from my solicitor – and please don't call on me for veterinary services in future. Goodbye.'

CHAPTER 39

Time for a Sabbatical

First of all I would go to the United States and visit my aunt in New York. Next it would be Uncle Fred in British Columbia.

Selling the business and property did not take long. I stayed on for a few weeks to introduce my successor, Dr Raine, a fine young married veterinarian who had been an assistant in a Newbury practice. His elderly father financed the purchase. Then I went up to my old stamping ground and stayed with my good friends, the Millers, at Mortimer. It was lambing time in early spring. I enjoyed the country atmosphere, the company of friends, the absence of telephone calls and not having the pressure of business.

Next I did locums in Upton-on-Severn where I met Members of Parliament Sir Anthony Eden and Sir Walter Monkton – and their dogs; then at Christchurch in the New Forest. Each place had better facilities than those available in my practice and I realized that the job could be made much easier by the expenditure of more money, both in equipment and staff. I should also add the benefits of a home and family impressed me when I visited other colleagues so blessed. I was filling in time while my application for entry to the United States as an immigrant was processed. Finally at the end of May I left Southampton Docks on a transatlantic liner.

My first trip across the 'ditch' to the United States was on the SS *Homeric*, owned by a German company and staffed mainly by Italians. There were a number of young people on board and before long we had pretty well found our niche. Since it was late spring, the seven-day crossing was reasonably calm. Table wine, first cousin to vinegar, was served at all meals. Beer had to be purchased. Fun and games and naughty nights made the passage very pleasant. On 2 July 1953, we persuaded the captain to put on a special event for the English passengers to celebrate Queen Elizabeth's coronation. A service was conducted by a German priest. This was followed by the ship's orchestra's interpretation of 'God Save the Queen'. They were half way through before we recognized the tune and stood up.

In New York I stayed for a time with my aunt Fan, my mother's elder sister, who had emigrated from England with her husband twenty years earlier. Their home was in Floral Park on Long Island. They had visited England with their two boys and a girl. We knew them well. My aunt, in a businesslike manner, had made appointments for me. My first was with Dr Garbutt who headed the ASPCA in a large animal hospital in the city. I watched him amputate a puppy's tail with scissors and collect $17.50 then we assembled in a tiered lecture room with several other veterinarians and a few nurses. An anaesthetised Border collie was carried in and placed on the demonstration table. Dr Garbutt addressed us. 'Today we have an interesting case of dislocated elbow. It doesn't happen often, fortunately, as it is difficult to get the joint back into normal position.' He heaved and tugged to replace the joint for ten minutes assisted by two brawny helpers until finally, after mopping his brow and straightening his tie, he confessed that this one was the most difficult he had encountered. He would have to do open surgery. Then he beamed at me and announced, 'We have an English doctor here today – let us see what he can do while I describe the surgery we will undertake.'

I went down to the table then quietly held the elbow joint in very tight flexion as I had done in many previous cases. For the next ten minutes the ligaments were stretched while I sat quietly. There were a few odd sniggers from the audience until, without any great effort, I repositioned the elbow joint with a loud click. Yes, I got applause. Later on Dr Garbutt complimented me, then offered a job at the hospital. But I didn't want to settle down and politely declined.

Two days later I was interviewed by the Chief Veterinarian at the Animal Health Department of New Jersey at Trenton. Again a job offer was turned down. The heat and humidity I found unbearable. After a week of family kindness and concern I announced my thanks and said I was packing a small carryall and would be heading north to cooler climes.

And so started an escape from organized endeavour plus an experience few people have an opportunity to enjoy in this world of conformity. I was going 'on the road'.

CHAPTER 40

Elmer Smith and Family

My 'on the road' adventure started with a Greyhound bus trip to Boston, which took a few hours. After arriving I found my way to the seafront where I rented a room for the night. I explored the city, leaving my meagre possessions, one change of underwear, two shirts, two pairs of socks, waterproof slicker, shaving gear and toothbrush in my room. As a seaport, Boston is a busy place. There is a large Irish element there. One story was repeated of the fellow who asked a passerby the quickest way to the hospital. He was told, 'Go into the nearest pub and shout "to hell with the Pope".'

My funds amounted to $100. Almost half of that was used up after some exciting entertainment at a nightclub called the Silver Dollar. A British naval warship was docked in the harbour on a courtesy visit. Several matelots had found their way to this lively nightspot. They were intrigued by the 'bar girls' who exhibited their shapely legs by dancing on the bar – above the pints and staring eyes. Next day I hoofed it out of town, stopping during a heavy downpour along with twenty or so other folks under a shop awning. I put my bag down by my feet where a small terrier dog sniffed around and cocked his leg on it. I lifted my foot and moved the little beast along, as I thought, quite gently.

A gruff voice sounded beside me, 'Whafo you kick ma dawg?' I turned to see a large irate black man, with eyes popping, who repeated the question in a more aggressive tone of voice. I then realized that the whole crowd was black and beginning to stare in my direction.

I said, 'I'm sorry, sir, but he was peeing on my bag.' I bent down ostensibly to show him but as soon as my hand grabbed the bag I pushed out of the crowd and, in spite of the rain, did the next one hundred yards in 'Bannister' time. Looking back, I was relieved to see they were not in hot pursuit.

By mid-afternoon I reached Highway 28, the main freeway going north. Traffic was rushing by at seventy miles an hour and was unlikely to stop for hitchhikers so I walked to the side expecting to come across a small town. By 6:00 p.m., footsore and tired, I found my way over a couple of fences to a farmhouse, which lay a quarter of a mile back from the highway. My knock on the front door was answered by a pleasant middle aged man. I said, 'I've walked about twenty-five miles today and am dead beat. If you need some help, could I sleep in the barn?'

He replied, 'Wait a minute,' then closed the door. Next, the door was opened by the farmer's wife.

She smiled and to my surprise – and great pleasure – said, 'We are just about to have supper. Would you like to have a hot bath first?'

My prayers were answered and I rapidly replied, 'You are very kind. I'd love to.'

After a hurried soak I joined the family at the large kitchen table. Farmer Elmer Smith, his wife, their parents, four teenagers and I sat down to a spread of ham, salad, home-made bread, strawberries and cream, lots of milk and a short prayer to go with it. Afterwards I was shown over to the barn which had steps leading up to a comfortable room which Smith told me had been occupied by an Italian prisoner of war who worked for them back in 1945. He dumped some bedclothes on the bed and asked if I could milk a cow.

'Done hundreds,' I lied – but that was to be my first job in the morning.

He had to shake me awake. 'I was calling you from downstairs for five minutes and thought you might have moved on,' he said. Then he took me down to a small cowshed and showed me a pail of warm water, a towel and a milk pail. 'Come over to the kitchen when you're done and we'll see about breakfast. Then we'll start getting the hay in if it's ready,' he told me.

Fortunately Bossy was a good-tempered Jersey and behaved herself while I dragged a gallon of milk from her.

Breakfast almost surpassed dinner and lunch was just as good. On this jaunt I used the name Harry. While Elmer and I harnessed the horse to the hay cart, his three Puerto Rican employees were working in the extensive market garden on the other side of the farmhouse. The hay had been collected into cocks. I pitched up to Elmer on the cart and he spread it around evenly until it was about to topple. Then we took it to the barn and forked it up into the loft. At the end of the third day my shoulders were aching but my feet were recuperating. We were finished with the hay.

I had enjoyed delicious meals and informative conversation when I told them I would be moving on the next day. Elmer said he could take me further north on Highway 28 as he was delivering fresh produce to a supermarket in Springfield. He handed me an envelope which I opened to see dollar bills inside.

'I didn't expect this when you so kindly took me on and really I feel I've been more than repaid for the work,' I stammered. He said I had earned it.

When he pulled the truck up to let me off he said, 'Harry, we needed some extra help for the hay but every year it's been difficult to get a good person. In a way we felt you had come at just the right time so both Mary and I thanked the good Lord for sending you.'

Such is faith – but I really can't take any credit.

CHAPTER 41

Portland

I was travelling north but still not far enough. My next ride was a good one, taking me to Portland in the State of Maine. The days were still hot and muggy. The thought of going to sea was appealing. Down near the docks I rented a sleeping room in a boarding house where a resident gave me a good lead. Mrs Maycroft needed someone to clean up a fish boat that had been out of commission for a couple of years. The family now hoped to put it back to work. A phone call put me in touch with the good lady who arranged that I would be picked up at 8:00 a.m. the following morning and given a day's work at $4.00 an hour.

Next morning a grizzled old sea dog drove me several miles to a rundown yard where what appeared to be an even more rundown boat, about forty-five feet long, rested on blocks. He left me with a bucket of lukewarm water, detergent and several rags, a tatty broom and three or four plastic garbage bags. 'I'll pick you up at five o'clock,' were his parting words.

I unlocked the cabin door and entered a scene of filth which is hard to describe. It seemed to be the dumping ground for old rope, old fish net, empty bottles, empty food cans, a few rags which had once been clothes, plus dirt, mould and cobwebs. Nevertheless by the end of the afternoon it was all spick and span though I was very much the worse for wear. The sea dog came back at five o'clock. Although we hadn't been introduced, I gathered he was the husband of Mrs Mycroft. He was anxious to get away but I insisted he inspect the results of my gruelling day's work without either food or drink, for there was no store nearby.

His attitude changed for the better. 'Listen young feller, there's a cook's job going on one of the wife's other boats. Have you ever done any cookin'?' he asked.

'Yes, I have,' came the quick reply, which wasn't a lie. I could remember warming up beans on toast at home, also putting raw spuds in a campfire when I was a boy scout. We drove over to a dock beside the Casco Bay Trading company, then he took me along the wharf where we came to a sixty-five foot vessel called the *Anna C* which was to be my home for a few weeks. 'What are you paying?' I asked.

He reached into his pocket and peeled off $36.00 which he gave me for my day's work. 'Now this will be different,' he explained. 'The boat is a gillnetter which leaves port at 1:00 a.m. with a captain and two crew. You will be catching cod and hake for the New York fresh fish market. Whatever it sells for, the owner gets fifty per cent, then there are five shares. The captain gets two and the rest is split three ways. You'll buy all your supplies and charge them to the *Anna C*. Now do you want the job?'

'Sounds good but let's go on board first,' I suggested. This we did. From the deck and down some steep steps the forecastle was roomy. It had two bunks on each side, one above the other. In the middle sat a table with a badly stained tablecloth. To one side was a wood stove with spring wires stretched across the top, some cupboards, a few wooden chairs and a head forward. 'Can I sleep aboard?' I asked.

'Yes you can,' he replied, 'but if you're going to eat the boat's grub you'll be docked fifteen a week.'

'Okay, I'll take it; when do I start?' I asked.

'They'll be coming aboard about 12:30 a.m. Just make sure you have breakfast ready for them,' he replied, then drove me back to my lodgings where I cleaned up and settled for five dollars as I was vacating the room early. It was 8:00 p.m. I had a hell of a lot to do.

CHAPTER 42

The Anna C

Back on the *Anna C* I was again cleaning up. The cupboards contained a variety of ancient plates, cutlery, cups – all heavily stained – plus packets of tea, coffee, sugar, milk powder and some cans of soup, fruit and vegetables. There was also a sink with one tap, a bottle of detergent and some rags. On the stove were a kettle, a cook pot and a large frying pan – not really the right setting for cordon bleu, but neither was the chef.

I went to the spacious Casco Bay Trading Company grocery store and identified myself as the new cook of the *Anna C*. The manager told me they hadn't had one for some time. Members of the crew were bringing their own food aboard every night. He had received a phone call confirming my authenticity and would be pleased to take care of my needs. He added, 'I'm told you're an Aussie. We haven't had many of them around for a while. Guess we're going to call you Digger.'

'You're right there mate,' I confirmed, and then went on a buying spree – tablecloth, dish towels, bread, bacon, butter, eggs, salt, pepper, jam, fruit cake, a couple of cantaloupes, a cooked chicken, some sliced ham, ketchup, paper towels, scrub brush and plastic plates. But that wasn't all. The bill came to $44.20 and I initialled it D.D. – A.C.

Back on board I ate a good meal, cleaned the stove, swept the floor, replaced the tablecloth and set three places at the table. There was electric light, one naked sixty-watt bulb. I made a mental note to go for a one hundred watt. A small portable radio blared western music as I prepared for my crew. Around midnight I lit the stove and had the kettle singing when Carl arrived. He was a tall middle aged Norwegian.

'I see you are making yourself at home then,' he said, with a heavy accent. Then he added, 'I had a phone call from Reg saying he had hired a cook. I'm the captain. Before long you'll meet Ernie and Jack. We're glad to have you. You'll give us breakfast when we leave the dock then dinner after we've hauled our net. I'll tell you the rest as we go along. That top bunk on the port side will be yours.'

Then the crew arrived. Ernie was short and stocky, more than middle aged, with the deep facial lines of a long time seafarer. Jack was much older, a North American Indian with a shock of white hair. Both grunted when I told them I was the new cook and my name was Digger. They sat at the table smoking while Carl had gone topside. I busied myself at the stove then after fifteen minutes placed before each of them a plateful of fried eggs, bacon, fried tomatoes, fried bread plus a cup of steaming coffee. Sugar, milk, pepper, salt ketchup and butter were presented in clean containers together with a paper napkin.

The 4000 hp diesel engine vibrated almost everything and before long we were under way. I kept Carl's meal warm. After a while Ernie got up and left to take over the wheel while the captain ate. There were no comments after the gargantuan meal – not until the third night.

It had been an exhausting day and more than half a night. After a brief clean-up I climbed into my bunk, a simple thing with gray bedclothes and pillow, which I discovered later had once been white. Next thing I knew I was being shaken by Jack and admonished in a gruff voice, 'Come on, cook – holidays are over.'

I scrambled out, very much aware of the ship's roll. Moving around the forecastle was difficult, at least until I found my sea legs several days later, by which time my side muscles ached from continual stretching.

A gillnetter catches fish by sinking a series of attached nets over a long distance. The net has a mesh with openings of four inches square. There are corks along one side and weights on the other. It is about four feet wide and sits on the ocean floor. When fish swim into it they can't reverse because the gills catch in the net. The one hundred yards or so of net are packed in open boxes placed on the deck. A marker buoy with eight-foot pole, carrying at its top tatters of what once were flags, identifies one end of the net's position, which is attached to its sinker. As the boat proceeds slowly forward the net is played out over the stern. When the end of the net is reached a second box is rapidly moved up and the new net tied to the one already put out. And so it goes on until eight or more nets have been set. Some are one-quarter mile in length in the general fishing area where a fairly level ocean bottom has been sought out by the skipper with his depth sounder. Finally, a second buoy is dropped to mark the far end of the net.

The following morning the buoy is located and the net hauled up. One side is secured around a wheel-like contraption which is turned by an engine, bringing the net in over the side and on to a table or bench. There the fish are removed and thrown into the spacious hold some twelve feet square and eight feet deep in the centre of the boat – like a large room.

My watch showed 5:30 a.m. We were out of sight of land. There were swells of about four feet but little wind. It was a clear day. The sun in the east was struggling for height. I was awed by the scene and felt very much at home, thinking that maybe I should have trained for the merchant marine service rather than vetting. The men of the crew were scanning the horizon for our buoy. It was soon spotted and we steamed over. Before long we had the net wrapped around the 'contraption' and had begun hauling. It was my job to control the speed at which the net came in. I was provided with a hammer to dispatch any dogfish accompanying the cod and hake. The catch was excellent and very few yards of net were hauled in without a good fish, some of which weighed around fifty or sixty pounds. The crew worked with gloves and the disentangled 'dogs' were thrown overboard. Some boats kept them and realized $10 a ton for export to Germany where apparently they were prized for fish and chips. A variety of fish and sea creatures came up and one day we had a five-foot long blue shark – which we threw back. Most of the fish were dead.

CHAPTER 43

In Command

On our return to port after the first day Carl asked me to come into the wheelhouse to learn how to run the boat. It was simple enough – wheel, throttle, forward and reverse, compass, light switch and windshield wipers. He even let me take over for five minutes while he went to the head. I felt good about it. On his return he said I should go to the Shamrock Bar and ask for Clem who would supply me with thigh boots and yellow oilskins for around $30. I presumed my duties had been performed satisfactorily and I was now part of the regular crew.

When we arrived back each day the first stop was near the harbour mouth where we unloaded the nets in open boxes at a big yard. Jack and I were left there to put the nets onto rotating frames then undo all the tangles. There was an elderly lady there who would repair any large tears.

Meanwhile the *Anna C* went over to the market area and unloaded the catch to be handled by our sales representative. When the boat returned, the boxes with folded nets were loaded on to the rear deck and we headed for our regular berth.

My day's work was done. It was about 3:00 p.m. First a swim off the dock then about five hours kip. I went to the market every evening to replenish supplies and pick up ice. Ernie brought a sack of wood and coal for the stove fire about every third night.

Then it was playtime, which was variously spent walking vigorously around the docks or at the Shamrock Bar where I fell in with some other ex-pats. One woman from Basingstoke had a comparable job as cook on a dragger, bigger than the *Anna C*, which went out for two weeks at a stretch. They were in port for the next four days. Maybe she would like to see my galley, I suggested.

The answer was yes. We had a lot in common and talked about things back home – but she insisted on taking my bedclothes to be laundered before she would share my bunk. I learned a lot more than cooking tips. She departed each night by 11:30 p.m., giving me time to prepare breakfast.

When I put the plate of fried food in front of Jack on the third night he hit the roof. 'What the hell are you doin' to us? Are you tryin' to kill us all? This god-damned fried food ain't good fer yer health.'

Maybe he was right. I said I'd boil him a couple of eggs, which he accepted. I realized my mistake and tried to provide a variety of more healthy fare, but breakfast is a tough one. Henry told me Carl wanted me in the wheelhouse so when I'd served him I went up.

We were heading down the estuary or wide inlet. On our port side was a string of buoys with lights to separate us from vessels heading into the docks. It was a clear night with little activity at that time. In the wheelhouse the only dim light was over the compass. Carl gave his orders.

'Take her down to the last of the lights. You'll know it because the end one is much bigger, then head her on a southeasterly course at sixteen degrees.' Then he left, leaving me in charge. I have been shortsighted since age fifteen and regularly wear specs, but on this trip I was experimenting to see if my eyesight would improve by not wearing them. They were in my bag by the bunk. A little prayer, a dose of cursing plus a lot of squinting and twenty minutes later we passed the last light. We were in the open sea travelling at better than fourteen knots. The Atlantic Ocean's swells were big but I found the right compass bearing. The only trouble was keeping her there. At that speed she seemed to yaw one way and when corrected went away out in the other direction. We travelled in a series of wide S's. I thought of Ernie's story about the prohibition days when they were making big money running booze down from Canada. The boat he was on was cut in two by a navy destroyer – both vessels running without lights. He was the only one saved out of a crew of four after eight hours in the water. But it didn't happen. When Carl came back about an hour later I wasn't more than ten degrees off our course. But later it took half an hour to locate our buoy even after radioing two other gillnetters in the vicinity for their assistance.

Some days, after a good catch, the hold was five feet deep in fish. Usually there was a rest period while I went below, lit the fire and put on dinner, which was served after we had set the new net. This dinner was to be my masterpiece: roast capon, potatoes, Brussels sprouts, yams, gravy and a tasty stuffing, all to be washed down with a bottle of beer.

I left it to cook in the oven while we set the new net. After I had dished up the meal we turned for home and while the other three went below to their magnificent repast I took the wheel. By this time I was an old hand and travelled a true and accurate course for dockside. Only a few minutes passed before Ernie was up in the wheelhouse and to my dismay reported, 'The chicken and the rest of it is half raw – still bloody.'

I asked him to take over the wheel then went below. The others were sitting back smoking while I re-stoked the fire which, for some reason, had not been drawing well. I opened the damper wide and told them, 'We'll gut the fish now then have dinner after we've done it.' They all agreed and while Carl took over the wheel the other two sharpened their knives. I dropped down into the hold, up to my waist or better in fish, and started to throw them up to the table, now some four feet above my head where the lads gutted them.

I used a three-pronged fork and, thanks to hay making, my muscles were up to it – except for the fifty-pounders which I implored the guys not to throw into the hold – but they took no notice. When the boat was rolling the last dozen or so were sliding all over the place and the cement floor was covered in slime. But I didn't break a leg and before long a hose was passed down to wash it all away

I had hardly climbed up the iron ladder to the deck when Jack shouted, 'We're on fire,' and it looked like it. Smoke was pouring from the forecastle hatch. I rushed down the steps and over to the stove and opened the oven door to reveal the source of the smoke. Jack was right behind me with a fire extinguisher. We gazed upon the blackened carcass of the capon, still emanating greasy smoke. Jack took one look and with the wisdom of an ancient Indian pronounced, 'Well, by Jesus, he's sure cooked now.'

CHAPTER 44

Shadow Bay Lodge

I was on the road again heading inland. The fishing was great but I wanted a change. I had cleared about fifty dollars a week but spent most of it. I left my oilskins and boots with Carl to sell then send me the cash at my New York address. I expected $35. It is still coming. I was fit, tanned, and full of vigour thanks to the healthy sea going experience.

Up through Bangor, after a succession of lifts, my next stop was Bar Harbor – the Capri of North America. I booked in for the night, not at the Marriott or the Hilton, but the Sally Anne – Salvation Army Hostel – in which the many cubicles were seven feet high in a large room with a ten-foot ceiling. The intervening spaces were wired in with some heavy mesh. Nighttime was a series of farts, grunts, retches and bronchial wheezes. But for $5 a night one can't be choosy.

It was the height of the tourist season. I soon had a job pulling beer in a very busy saloon which employed four waitresses kept constantly on the move. In between table service they put on the 'girlie' floorshow.

After the bar closed at 1:00 a.m. I joined a bunch of merrymakers in the street where we sang 'Red River Valley' and a few other favourites. It didn't please the local police chief who arrived with three burly henchmen and threatened a bunk in the hoosegow if we didn't shut up. I spent another night with the grunts.

In the morning I collected my one day's pay of $25 then headed for Saratoga Springs, the famous horse racing city. It was off season and not worth hanging around.

A few miles hitching took me to the State Capital, Albany. I was using up my meagre funds so felt another residential job would take care of things – and it did. At an employment agency I bargained away half of my first week's wages but I had a job. Shadow Bay Lodge on Lake George needed a dishwasher. We were in the second week of August. At that time it was very difficult to find a replacement for the one who had quit. I learned later, to my cost, that the sink was lower than regulation and the cause of many sore backs in otherwise willing workers. It took me the best part of the day to get there.

It was 8:00 p.m. as I headed off the main road and down a long driveway to the lodge, which consisted of a main central building and various cabins stretched along the shore. It was a beautiful setting.

One of the cabin boys took me in hand and showed me up to the dormitory above the kitchen. He indicated a bed the previous dishwasher had used which he hoped would suit me. Then he added, 'We were expecting you earlier. The dishes will be piling up from the dining room. You're expected to start right away.'

He led me down to the kitchen and introduced me to Danny who was to be my helper, a good little chap of some sixteen years who had already filled the two large adjoining sinks with hot water. The right one was given some detergent and the left a dash of Chloros.

The soiled plates, glasses and cutlery were brought from the dining room by the waiters and placed on a large table to my right. Danny sorted them out, throwing the leftovers into the garbage, then I took over. The hardest part was bending over the low sinks. After washing, things were put into the very hot left sink for a couple of minutes and then up on racks to dry. This also was Danny's job. We slaved for over two hours until the dishes arrived in smaller quantities. Some rotten sods sat in there until well after 11:00 p.m. before relinquishing their plates.

It had been a long day. Bed was welcome and in spite of sharp little pains in my back, sleep soon took over.

Most of the staff were university students, males unfortunately. The cook was older while his adolescent son was a busboy. Clem was the headwaiter with three assistants. Two more were cabin cleaners and John took care of the assortment of boats at the dock.

CHAPTER 45

Melanie

The routine put me at the sink around 9:00 a.m. when the breakfast dishes began to pile up. Late risers tended to prolong the operation but usually by 11:30 a.m. I could get away for a swim in the lake. Same routine after lunch and then a good break until around 7:00 p.m. which was the busiest time of all. In the afternoon break, and often in the early morning the cook's son, Frank, and I would take a canoe and go fishing for bass with excellent results.

After two days at the sink my back was so sore it was all I could do to reach the stairs, go up to the dormitory, and lie down on my bunk until called back to the sink by Danny. The owner's wife, who hosted the cocktail hour, came out to the kitchen at the start of the evening shift.

'Harry,' she said, 'we have some leftovers which might help your back,' as she placed a cocktail shaker one-third full of Martini on the bench. It did – and became a nightly routine.

One afternoon when out in the canoe I saw a very attractive blonde woman on the shore and waved to her. She waved back. Next day she was there again and as we went near I told Frank to come back in half an hour then I jumped overboard and swam ashore. Melanie was in her late teens, a beautiful figure in a white one-piece bathing costume, with a lovely face and friendly smile. She told me she was up at the lake at their summer home but usually resided in Kentucky where her father, a vice president of Sonocan Electric, raised racehorses. She had been attending finishing school in Maryland.

We met daily, chatted about life in general and swam together. She only saw me in bathing trunks. I told her I was staying at the Lodge. On about the fourth meeting she produced a little hand drawn map of how to reach her house by road and invited me to come for dinner on the following Sunday evening – and meet her parents.

I had two days to prepare for the visit. The cook loaned me a respectable suit. Henry Alcan, the owner, had a shirt and tie I could borrow. Clem had socks and shoes that would fit and Bill Myers offered to man the sink on Sunday evening – for $10. At the appointed time Henry drove me in his Cadillac over to my date, leaving the main road then passing through fully one-quarter of a mile of beautiful parkland. We reached a large, rambling, Tudor style home, surrounded by well tended flower beds, a couple of statues, a large pond and a couple of tennis courts. Henry dumped me off and I headed for the front door, which was opened by a uniformed butler and Melanie. We went into a large lounge overlooking the lake about one hundred yards away. I was introduced to her folks and her brother. The 'old man' was in his sixties, I estimated: a youthful figure, upright stance, shock of white hair and large similarly coloured moustache. His main feature was a pair of piercing eyes which seemingly already accused me of raping his daughter – which I hadn't. His wife was a lovely person exuding friendly conversation which made me feel at home. (Are you kidding?) Her brother was about fourteen and quite mature.

We looked at her yearbook from school, each student given a full page with photograph plus list of attributes. But there was no Martini or scotch and I learned later that both alcohol and nicotine were banned. Dinner in an oak-paneled dining room was served by the butler. A uniformed maid whose main duty was refilling the ice water glasses also helped.

After the meal Melanie and her brother took me to a recreation room where we played table tennis then rummy. I didn't see her folks again. They had learned from me that I was indeed a fully qualified veterinarian who had come out from the UK to do research with a major pharmaceutical company called Merck, Sharpe and Dohme in New York. I had flown up to the Lodge for a short holiday.

I asked Melanie if I could take her to see a movie on the following Wednesday. She was doubtful but would ask her parents. Then, accompanied by her brother, she drove me back to the Lodge. I was to phone on Tuesday morning at exactly 11:00 a.m., which I did, and was delighted by her excitement that permission was granted but William would have to come along too as chaperon.

They picked me up at 7:00 p.m. on Wednesday in the family Caddy then off we went to Glen Falls, some seven miles away. The movie house was comfortable in the back row. While William went out to the snack bar to spend the several dollars I handed him in the course of the main feature, Melanie surrendered herself to my kisses and responded with a fire that portended many treats ahead. All I got when she dropped me off at the Lodge was a peck on the cheek which I am sure would be reported to Daddy by the chaperon.

When I telephoned next morning at 11:00 a.m. the call was answered by the butler. 'Miss Melanie has returned to Kentucky to get ready for the next school term.'

And so ended a beautiful, if brief, romance.

CHAPTER 46

Kitchen and Island High Jinks

A large table was set aside in the spacious kitchen where the staff took their meals on a somewhat irregular basis according to the demands of their duties. The fare was excellent. In addition, many extras came my way after the trays were brought out from the guest dining room: T-bone steaks from which a square inch had been cut from the centre, untouched lobster tail with melted butter, and half full bottles of wine. All the goodies were put on the shelf to be taken up to the dormitory after my shift for the benefit of the other staff.

Bill Myers was a cabin boy, a serious type of youth who normally attended bible college and was now hoping to raise some finances for the coming year. One evening after an early finish at the sink we walked up to the highway and thumbed a ride to Glen Falls, a resort town on the shore of Lake George. Next, it was into one of the many saloons where the holiday crowd was in high spirits well maintained by an excellent piano player. There was some desultory singing by less inhibited singers. Then, after the third glass of beer, I gave a rendering of *When Irish Eyes are Smiling* which was well received. A waiter delivered several more glasses of beer to our table with the compliments of appreciative patrons. This prompted me to renderings of *Galway Bay, Colonial Boy* and a few others.

By midnight singing was out of the question and standing difficult. Bill Myers was asleep at another table using his folded arms as a headrest. He became quite hostile when I tried to rouse him for the homeward trek. The journey back to the Lodge was a nightmare, with Bill throwing himself down on the roadway while I had to pull him out of the path of approaching cars, which fortunately were not frequent. He also had a tendency to burst into song though his repertoire didn't go much beyond 'Rock of Ages' and 'Jesus Loves Me'.

The dawn was showing up in the distant east when I pushed a sobering Bill up the stairs, then, fully clothed, into his bed. His shift as a cabin boy wouldn't start until 11:00 a.m. I resolved not to take

Bill pubbing again. Clem came instead and we enjoyed free beer whenever I was persuaded to exhibit my baritone – or was it tenor – on Irish ballads.

One evening in the pub we met a Welshman called Evan Porter who had joined in the rendering of 'Danny Boy'. He was a waiter at a local holiday resort called 'The Island', which it was. It could only be reached across a bridge manned by uniformed security guards to ensure that only registered guests were admitted. Not knowing who we were or where we came from he said if ever we came to one of their Saturday night dances, which were open to the public, he would take care of us – and he did.

One of our Lodge rules was that staff were not allowed to use the motor boats. To get a key for the boathouse from John, the boat boy, it took a lot of persuasion and an undertaking not to start the engine until we were two hundred yards away. On a Saturday night after work four of us, Bill Myers (in spite of my resolution), Frank, the cook's son, Clem and I headed into the gathering dusk towards 'The Island'. It was 11:00 p.m. when we reached there and pulled the boat up the beach on the dark side of the island. There was no difficulty finding the action. Before long we were in the main dance hall flirting with the many lovely ladies who, possibly encouraged by several gin and tonics, were literally letting their hair down. We found seats at a table with three other couples. We asked if Evan Porter was around, but he had spotted us and brought over four beers and a plate of sandwiches. We introduced ourselves with fictitious names and joined in the dancing and merrymaking until it ended at 1:00 a.m.

We had no trouble finding our boat. The journey back to the Lodge had its moments. We could not see very much as most of the shore lights were out at that time. There was little moonlight, often obscured by fleeting clouds. Bill Myers felt we were not chugging fast enough with the small outboard motor so took the oars and began rowing at a frantic pace. I imagine the rest of us were too tired to do anything about it until he fell over backwards with his feet in the air and holding on to only one oar. We searched around for half an hour but never found the left one. It made paddling into the dock more difficult but by that time the first glimmer of dawn helped.

Again I resolved not to take Bill Myers pubbing.

CHAPTER 47

End of the Big Adventure

The pace of life was hectic. Not the job, but the after hours 'goings on', or shall we kindly call it recreation. My young fellow workers were a good cross section of American youth. I found them friendly, co-operative, witty, and talented. I liked them all. My boss, Henry Alcan, was a very fair, generous person who was always ready to give a word of encouragement. Mrs Alcan was thoughtful and I really think her 'gin gesture' made it possible for me to continue in the job. It was also my happiest escape from the routines and pressures of professional life. But it was to end soon. Closing date for the season was Labour Day, the first Monday in September. For me it was back to New York by Greyhound bus with $74.00 to show for my various labours. The next chapter in my prolonged holiday was about to begin with a return to respectability.

My aunt and family were shocked at the well censored stories I told of my exploits, feeling that my time should be spent in pursuing a more conventional occupation which would also be more rewarding financially. I agreed, then announced that I would be going to Cleveland to visit my old friend from the Reading days, Dr David Rickards. He had left the UK a few years earlier, then, after several assistant jobs, had set up his own office which he named 'Small Animal Clinic'. Many of his clients called him Dr Small – which I did whenever I phoned him. It was a confusing name. In the course of time he met several potential clients who had taken their great Danes to other vets.

There was another side to the story, which Rick told me: 'A middle aged lady used to bring her dog to me and I was lucky because it got over some obscure disease for reasons which are beyond my ken. The lady was delighted and wanted to impress me.

'"Young man," she said as she stood by the front door, "I want to tell you what a good job you did. I have been coming in here for years," she went on (which was a lie because we had only opened the year before), "and I know the owner, Dr Small, very well.

Next time I see him I'm going to tell him what a good doctor you are."

' "Thank you so much," I replied. "Maybe the old skinflint will give me a raise." '

CHAPTER 48

Cleveland, Ohio

The bus trip took most of the day and it was early evening when Rick met me then took me to his clinic on Euclid Avenue. It was a large store in a busy shopping centre which had been remodelled to his requirements. While he treated his patients I was directed to a used car sales lot, not far away, to pick out something suitable but cheap. Happily my aunt had boosted my finances with money sent out, I believe against regulations, by my mother. I didn't rush into any deal.

It took me two hours of horse-trading and $750 to acquire a 1942 Ford. I was not familiar with the methods of the salesman, who couldn't conclude a deal without approval of his manager – who was out to supper for thirty minutes at a time. The price on the car's windscreen read $950 and it came down about $25 a time after which the manager had to be consulted while I sat in their uncomfortable waiting room. Finally my offer of $750 was accepted. Yes, they were losing money.

After all the papers were signed there was a ten-minute wait while they ensured that the car's oil, gas and water were topped up. Then I drove over to the clinic where Rick was concluding his evening consulting. When we left half an hour later, my excitement was dulled as I saw a rapidly expanding pool of water spreading under the front wheels. I had been suckered or swindled – or both. Rick thought it a minor problem. Surprisingly, a can of 'stop leak' poured into the radiator effected a permanent repair.

Rick was married to a lovely lady, Marjory. They had a very young daughter, Barbara Susan. They lived in a fourth floor apartment in Shaker Heights, a fashionable area. The city was very cosmopolitan with national and linguistic areas of blacks, Italians, Dutch and Orientals. It was also an area of heavy industry and frequent crime. Business was moving out of the downtown to the suburbs. A lot needed to be done. Fortunately, an efficient city administration spent millions, rapid transit was built and fashionable areas developed so that when I went back for a visit twenty years later it was delightful.

I was invited to stay at their apartment. It was early winter. The steam heat central heating bothered me. Rick took a hammer and started bashing the pipes. He then phoned down to the janitor to tell him there was an air lock in the system so he would have to reduce the heat. It worked and comfort returned.

A move was coming up to a country house where they would share with another person, although the accommodation itself was separate. One problem was to move a very large and long settee which had been built in the apartment by a previous tenant. They had inherited it when they moved in. It had been my bed for a few weeks. It could go down neither the elevator nor stairways. Undaunted, we rented a heavy block and tackle with a really long rope then put our knot tying knowledge to work. It also necessitated removing the entire window frame.

After a couple of hours work on a Sunday morning the 'thing' sat on a rented truck and was triumphantly hauled away to its new home. But don't think the problem was solved. From the new hallway it couldn't be turned into any of the downstairs rooms. On the second floor there was nowhere on which to hang the block. With some sharp scissor work from Marge and a borrowed saw from the neighbour we divided it into equal halves which solved the problem of getting it into the downstairs lounge. Putting it together again worked well until the evening when guests from the prestigious Cleveland Clinic came to dinner. Doctor Mathias, a 200-pounder from the pathology department, ensconced himself on the settee together with the thin-as-a-rail admissions secretary. As we all enjoyed a hearty laugh the damned thing collapsed in the middle, throwing her on top of him. We were laughing so much it took five minutes to untangle them.

Rick is a very intelligent and interesting character. His father was a well-known businessman in the London rag trade who I met a few years later when he insisted on giving my pregnant wife a maternity dress. Among other things Rick is a Humanist. This is not a creed well known in the UK, but essentially, its followers decry the established ecclesiastical dogma and believe that peace of mind and spirit depend on your own efforts to live the good life. They are unnecessarily critical of other beliefs. Rick wrote many letters to the

126

Cleveland Plain Dealer on the subject under the pseudonym A.T. Heist. The many people who commented and replied to Mr Heist's views did not appreciate the significance of 'atheist'.

He was also a knowledgeable astronomer. Together we spent many interesting times scanning the heavens through his telescope. We played golf at one of Cleveland's most fashionable courses where ladies' skirts could not come above the knee. It was compulsory to employ a caddy at a cost of $5 a round. At the first green and out of sight of the clubhouse each one was given a dollar then sent back. At the end of the round in the men's locker room we ordered drinks which were prepared while we showered, slippers and towels provided, after which we leisurely dressed, our suits having been pressed and shoes polished by the negro called Sam.

We went night clubbing together with Marge and a friend. We enjoyed the best seats. Good meals and drinks came with excellent service. Rick refused my willingness to contribute to the bill. I learned later that Marge was a roving reporter for the national magazine *Billboard*. Her presence at any nightclub might produce a favourable mention in its columns, which would be publicity one couldn't buy. Hence, no bill.

I met several interesting people. The Rickards had a wide circle of friends, many from the Cleveland Clinic. I stayed for a week with the Grundish family out at Gates Mills. Roger Grundish was a very competent and well-known veterinarian, the only one I ever saw who conducted his evening clinic while smoking a large cigar. I always think of him when I see on television a professional golfer with a stogie in his mouth while trying to line up a putt. After a few days as we sat in his comfortable lounge in the evening, he remarked to his wife, Beth, 'You can put the books back now.' It was explained that Roger had meticulously scanned his bookshelves for any material of a political nature or off beat philosophy. This was an example of the mania sweeping America before McCarthyism was exposed by the US army brass as being a character-destroying persecution worse than the communism it purported to demean.

I did a locum for two weeks while a friend of Rick's took a vacation. I enjoyed it although I was not really licensed to do it. One of Rick's previous jobs was at Aurora with Dr Dykstra. He suggested I go out there and visit him, which would take me some twenty-five miles west of Chicago. A phone call from Rick assured me of a warm welcome.

Urolithiasis is a medical term for stones or mineral crystals in the urine of a patient. It surprised me when I first came to Cleveland in 1953 that it had become a troublesome condition in neutered male cats, many of whom could not be cured, necessitating prolonged medication and sometimes euthanasia.

Part of the problem was felt to be due to early neutering of male cats which had not reached sexual maturity. The sexual organs, particularly the penis, would be in an undeveloped state with a narrow urethra, which is the passageway through which the urine is voided. The crystals in their early stages and small size could be passed but when a number were clumped together in a hard mass passage was impossible. Urine accumulated in the bladder causing initially pain and distress but before long uremia followed by death.

Dr Rickards' investigation sought out a dietary cause. Before long he determined that nearly all of the cases he had treated were being fed almost exclusively on a popular canned cat food consisting of cooked ground-up fish – bones and all. It was at this time that the small herring-like fish off South America were being netted by the thousands of tons with no major human market. Could there be a connection?

A compilation of his case histories was sent to the manufacturer of the food with his conclusion that the high mineral content of their canned cat food contributed to the feline problem in over 87 per cent of cases he had treated.

The reply came a few weeks later. 'Your records should also be checked for broken legs. You will not be surprised that 87 per cent of all such cases are also being fed the same diet. Are you suggesting the diet is also responsible for these?'

Dr Rickards spread the word of his convictions among his clients and also developed a technique for the surgical treatment of the condition which he called the 'Cleveland Technique'. It was widely acclaimed in the veterinary press.

In the course of time and after many research experiments had proved the cause of the condition to be dietary, cat diets were altered to eliminate certain minerals with the happy result that the condition is now a rarity.

CHAPTER 49

Dr Merrick and Aurora

The Ford travelled well on the busy highways. My first overnight was Chicago on the shores of Lake Michigan. Driving around the city to see the sights, I found myself on the 'Loop', skirting the busy downtown while following the lakeshore. Traffic was six abreast, hurtling along at sixty miles an hour. I was fully five miles out of the city before it was safe to change lanes and find a way off. I drove back to the downtown then parked the car by driving through what looked like a gutted store but led into a labyrinth of parking spaces six stories high and more than one hundred yards long. It cost me ten dollars for overnight parking which is what I paid for my own accommodation in a rundown wino's hotel not far away.

My next quest was to find the veterinary hospital of Dr Andy Merrick, a legend amongst his colleagues, who had greatly impressed Dr Rickards. He received me heartily. I learned that Rick had phoned him that morning, 'To expect a visit from a prominent member of the profession in the UK.'

Andy was probably in his late sixties. He had been in this downtown practice for thirty years. He had many innovative ideas. I learned from Rick that he had developed a formula for a lotion that was very effective in treating eczema in dogs, which was, and is, a common complaint often associated with flea infestation – but not always. He wanted to sell the product commercially, having had several thousands of six-ounce bottles already made up. He was unable to find any pharmacy willing to handle it. He put a half page advertisement in the *Chicago Tribune*: 'Dr Merrick's wonder cure for dog eczema. You can now clear up this troublesome complaint by using a daily application of Scratchex, obtainable from Sears Roebuck and Myer's Pharmacy.' Neither had heard of Merrick but were the largest medicine dispensers in the city. Before long Andy's phone was ringing off the hook as the store managers frantically sought a supply of the wonder lotion to meet the demands of their many dog-owning customers. Within months the medication was obtainable throughout the United States. I believe it is still an often-used very effective medication – and I expect ensured a comfortable retirement for Andy.

After being shown around his busy hospital we adjourned to his office for some refreshment. I told him I was very impressed with the facility but I noticed that he had no X-ray equipment. I doubted whether one could diagnose certain fractures or foreign bodies without it. Andy held up his left hand from which I noticed three fingers missing. 'This is what X-ray has done for me,' said Andy, 'and many other doctors who have lost all their fingers, now forced into retirement or old folks' homes.' Then he added the classic comment, 'They'll shit – if somebody feeds them.'

It was so true of the early use of X-rays in diagnosis. Professionals later learned that irreversible damage to living tissue could result from not wearing protective clothing and lead-lined gloves while using it. He now referred all X-ray work to another hospital on a fee-splitting basis, the diagnostic films and the patient being subsequently returned to his office

I was very impressed with the handling of traffic by the Chicago police. There were several one way streets on which traffic might be travelling six abreast during rush hour. At the intersections were traffic lights. There was a small raised island in the centre with a policeman following the light changes with the loud blowing of a whistle plus arm waving to either move the traffic along or stop it in an orderly manner. There was no pushing into the intersection on the amber light such as I see in Vancouver where our gendarmes prefer to wait around the corner to hand out a ticket rather than expose themselves and assist the traffic flow.

Next day it was on to Aurora, a pleasant town of some forty thousand people. I rented a cheap room then drove out to Dr Dykstra's veterinary hospital. It had been purpose built, with plenty of parking, plus well-tended planters of shrubbery. Inside was a waiting room for dogs and one for cats, which in those days was very innovative. The rest of the layout was modern and efficient, as were the numerous nurses and other staff. Dyk was essentially a large animal practitioner who wore white pants and jacket on his rounds. A middle-aged assistant took care of the small animal side of the practice. I should add here that in those days veterinarians worked a very full day with offices open from 8:00 a.m. until 8:00 p.m., snatching an odd half hour for a bite to eat but not reaching home for a good dinner until late evening.

The hospital had its own X-ray technician. Garry Langston was a great character. During the thirties he had served with Claire Chennault and the Flying Tigers in China. He was full of stories about their exploits.

It seemed unnecessary to have such a person in a small animal hospital until I learned that he also did other things. His machine, a portable X-ray, was low-powered – something like thirty-five amps – though I am not too familiar with the details. He asked me if I would like to go to the 'track' and assist him in his horse therapies. We went one morning to the Chicago Trotting Raceway which was a journey of twenty miles. Associated with all tracks are countless loose boxes for stabling the horses plus walking and washing areas. We set up his X-ray in a loose box and before long had a queue of horses lined up for treatment. Each horse was individually brought in and held by its halter by the stableman while Garry positioned his X-ray about twenty inches from behind the front legs with the aperture directed at the tendons. When he switched on there was a buzzing sound. Each leg was given a thirty-second 'Ray Spray'. The horse was led out for the next one to come in. On that morning seven horses had lined up. In all sincerity Garry told me that he had instituted the procedure about ten months previously with the permission of Dr Dykstra on an experimental basis. Surprisingly, trainers taking advantage of this new, and as yet unheard of, therapy, claimed to have had more winners than ever before. At ten dollars a session it had paid good dividends. I was sceptical and suggested to Dr Dykstra that this was charlatanism and unethical. He said it was experimental and on trial. He had spoken to several trainers who wanted to continue.

He also told me of a case in a cow with actinomycosis or 'lumpy jaw'. After failing to cure the condition with repeated injections of sodium iodide intravenously, he had asked Garry to try X-ray therapy. Surprisingly, after four treatments spaced about one week apart, the mass of diseased tissue had regressed and almost disappeared. But I am still sceptical.

Dr Dykstra was the track veterinarian. In the evening his duties included taking samples from the first and second horse after each race plus any others when the stewards requested it. I went with him

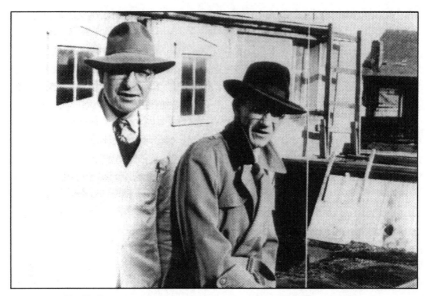

Dr Dykstra and Garry Langston, Aurora, Illinois, USA.

one evening. We arrived at the track around 5:30 p.m. After parking
the car in a designated space, we went to the clubhouse for a drink
and light meal, which was fairly rushed as we had to be on duty at
6:00 p.m. when the first race was run. Dyk told me we would not go
back to the clubhouse or the betting areas until we had completed
the evening's work. When the two subject horses were brought in to
the testing barn, which was open to the public who stood behind a
rail, each was backed into a stall. A metal syringe with four-inch
nozzle was pushed into the mouth and four ounces of white vinegar
squirted in. The profuse salivation was collected in a large enamel
dish then emptied into two six-ounce jars. These were capped with a
screwed metal cover and a label was attached over the top then down
each side, identifying the horse, the race location and the time, plus
the name of the owner and trainer. One jar was given to the trainer.
The other would be sent to the State Gaming Laboratory for drug
testing. In some cases a urine sample was requested by the Race
Committee which became more difficult. In mares a slice of raw
onion was inserted into the vagina which invariably produced rapid
co-operation. For males there was a stableman who had a peculiar
whistling ability which, when continued for a couple of minutes,
was successful in producing a flow. For those not musically inclined,

or perhaps deaf, a stable boy holding a can on a long pole under-neath the belly entailed a prolonged wait sometimes lasting several hours after racing ceased. When we were finished our duties, which was usually around 11:00 p.m., a policeman would escort us to our car.

My ten-day visit was most enjoyable. The hospitality I received both at the Dykstras and at several farmhouses was appreciated, particularly as my humble accommodation in mid-winter was not very comfortable.

CHAPTER 50

Seeing the Hopkinsons
– and Tying the Knot

It was late winter in Cleveland – cold, snowy, and miserable. Returning from my visit to Aurora I spent a few days with the Rickards before fulfilling a commitment I had made a year or two earlier to visit the Hopkinsons in Ontario. I picked a bad time to travel. On the Queen Elizabeth Highway heading to Toronto it was snowing lightly. I pushed on with foot hard down on the gas pedal, conscious of the weaving of the car, which I attributed to ice on the roadway. When I pulled in to refuel I found the left rear tire flat almost to the rim. I had the spare put on.

Overnight in Toronto was not very impressive. It was not the best time to appreciate its beauty. Next day, on to MacDonald's Corners where all the roads were snow-covered. I couldn't get up even small hills and went into a couple of farms for help. Fortunately, each one had a contract to sand the road surface when requested – but they cursed me for not having snow tires. Later on I put some heavy cases of dog food into the trunk which helped with the traction. Following the farmers' directions I drove several miles into a more desolate wooded area with no farms or buildings. I saw the sign, 'Little Rapids House' and underneath 'Uxmore Kennels'. I turned into a long driveway which took me to a lovely house overlooking a river now partially covered with ice and snow. Peter and Jo greeted me warmly. The dozen or so corgis milled around, fortunately not yapping as they had the last time I had seen them. After a few drinks and lunch we sat in the lounge before a roaring fire and caught up with each other's news. Peter had by this time been recognized as a first class judge of dogs, presumably by winning so many trophies with the corgis, of which several of the original purchase remained. He had been invited to judge three classes at the Westminster Show to be held in New York in mid March, indeed a great honour.

The days passed happily, feeding and brushing the dogs, all of which lived inside the house at this time of year, the temperature often being 30 degrees below freezing at night. The dogs enjoyed frolicking in the snow following their daily walks over the property. According to naval tradition we never 'indulged' before noon, at which time a couple of gin and tonics made the lunchtime conversation more sparkling. Peter had many reminiscences of his naval career, Jo had been a racing car driver, and, well, I always had a fistful of yarns.

We made several trips into Perth where Peter was greeted warmly by the trades people we met when picking up supplies. The Canadian scene appealed to me. I became interested in learning about its history, a stormy beginning which had potential for unrest in later years. I also read the poems written by Robert Service about the life and hardships in the Yukon. One evening while a snowstorm raged outside we sat in front of a blazing fire in the lounge where I wrote 'The Trapper's Friend' in a similar idiom. Here it is:

The Trapper's Friend
'E follered me back from the trading post
And squatted outside the shack;
An' 'e sat there most of the next day too
An' showed no sign o' goin' back.
'E wasn't no prize or any known breed
An' nothin' about 'im was neat,
But 'e wagged 'is tail and barked for joy
When I wrassled some grub to eat.
Now I'm not a man who's fond of dogs
But somethin' about that stray
Touched me inside 'cos 'e'd come to me
An' showed me 'e wanted to stay.
'E'd 'ad a rough time I knew for sure
For 'e cowed when I told 'im what for
An' 'e wouldn't follow me down to the post,
But stayed at the shack by the door.
Now I never did 'ear who owned 'im afore,
An' I never let on where 'e was
But 'e let me know 'e'd settled right down
And moved inside like in-laws.
Soon everthin's jake 'tween 'im and me,
And no one comes near anyway,

135

But if 'e was priced at a thousand bucks
I know I'd fork out so 'e'd stay.
Yes, stupid you'll think amongst all yer pals
An' plenty of laughs would arise,
But up in the wilds you're out o' this world
An' live lonely and comfortless lives.
A lick of 'is tongue or a laugh in 'is eyes
An' you're workin' away with a grin,
An' no backchat or arguments
To wear your temper thin.
But that's a few summers and winters past
An' many a trap line I've walked,
With 'im at me 'eels a waggin' 'is bush
Or barkin' replies as we talked.
We've been shacked up for weeks on end
While a blizzard covered the trail,
But nary a question or grumble came
From 'im as 'e wagged 'is tail.
'E'd share me grub an' 'e'd lick the plates
An' 'e'd catch them pack rats too
An' 'e'd lie at the foot of me rough hewn bed
An' sleep the long nights through.
'E saved me life, an' I'll swear to that
When we ran in dutch with a bear,
For 'e stood 'is ground and bared 'is teeth
An' gave me time to get clear.
An' once when the booze 'ad bested me
I lay 'alf numbed in the snows,
But 'e got me round and sobered me up
By pushin' me face with 'is nose.
'E's shared me life and I've shared 'is
But it wasn't no ordeal.
I couldn't 'ave asked for a truer friend
Or a love that was 'alf as real.
Three score and ten is a ripe old age
So I'm knockin' on the door,
And the cur is greyed and slowed in step
An' 'ardly goes out any more.
But if 'e could foller me up to them gates

St Peter might let 'im slide by
For all that I'd ask in the heaven above
Was to be with that dear old guy.

But there is a limit, so after three weeks I felt it was time to move on. It was desolate country and I had a lot of travelling to do before settling down.

One evening Peter said, 'Ernie, you know we will be away for about ten days at the show. Would you consider staying on and taking care of things here?'

It would be in three weeks time. I thought a bit and finally replied, 'Yes, I would, Peter, but I'm going to make a strange request. I would like to propose marriage to June and ask her to fly out here so that we could marry before moving on.' They were delighted. They had never met her but had known that after being my head nurse back in the UK we had a strong affection for each other.

Over the next few weeks we all enjoyed talking about the approaching nuptials. Peter's ribald jokes were an embarrassment for Jo. When my proposal was accepted June was working at a veterinary clinic in London. She was excited at the prospect and booked a flight to Montreal for 14 March. At my end I had to have banns read at the local parish church. I found, after much searching, a clergyman who would come to the house to perform the ceremony. The Reverend Campbell at Lanark was a delightful person, tall, with flowing white hair, now retired from regular duties. When I made my request he said the fee would be three dollars. I told him I wasn't religious but had been to Sunday school as a child. Church attendance was mandatory at boarding school, twice daily, which is probably the reason I was disenchanted. I said I didn't want anything beyond the minimum, no bowing and scraping.

The reverend admonished me. 'Young man, you do not kneel to me but to your maker.' It cut me down to size. I picked 16 March for the wedding when my hosts would be departing to New York. The ceremony was to take place in their lounge. Peter warned me not to look down as Campbell had the biggest feet in Canada – size fourteen shoes, which had to be specially made.

I drove up to Montreal on the morning of 14 March, expecting to meet June off the plane around 4:00 p.m. then drive back. The plane was delayed until the following morning. I persuaded Air Canada that a night's accommodation plus meal vouchers were the least they could do for me. I spent a pleasant evening with others in the same predicament. June arrived the next morning, complete with fur coat, looking very charming. When we arrived at Perth it was 2:00 p.m. on a Wednesday. As the shops were closed, I couldn't buy a ring. Back at the house Jo said we could borrow hers. June was to occupy a bedroom next to mine. Peter told me a regular check would be made through the night to ensure there were no premature try-outs. Peter told June he was surprised her parents had given consent for such an innocent, sweet, young child to marry an old reprobate like me. At the time June was twenty-one and I was ten years her senior.

On the morning of 16 March, Campbell duly arrived at 11:00 a.m. We stood before him and took our vows, while Peter repeatedly pointed down so that I would see the big feet. I was almost in hysterics. When it came to putting on the ring it didn't fit. I had a hard time containing myself. Afterwards we had some bubbly and cake and signed some papers; I paid Campbell the three dollars, we took some photographs, then he left. A light meal was served, the Hopkinsons departed, and my honeymoon commenced.

For the next ten years I sent the Reverend Campbell $10 every Christmas with my current address. He reminded me where he was by sending a card in the first week of December. The last one came from an old folks' home somewhere, and then there were no more.

When Jo and Peter got back I told them that we would be on our way, first to visit my aunt in New York, then an old uncle in British Columbia. It embarrassed me to tell Peter I was broke and could he lend me a couple of hundred until my annual remittance arrived in June. This he readily did. We departed in a blizzard, winter's final kick, crossing into the US at Buffalo after an hour's haggling with the immigration officer. Next morning there were twenty-five inches of snow on the ground. Schools were closed with most transport at a standstill. My car licence had expired and now I had a wife to support! June saved the day by admitting her mother had hidden several large banknotes in the lining of her fur coat. For a while my troubles were solved. As there had been some doubt that June would be permitted entry to the US I wired Peter, 'It's a fine day in the USA.'

CHAPTER 51

Married and in the US Again – and Uncle Fred

By mid-day the roads were clear and we started on our way to Cleveland. The good old Ford behaved well. Our first priority was to renew the licence. We stayed with the Rickards for a few days then drove via the Pennsylvania Turnpike down to New York City. It was an excellent highway. The mileage was recorded where you got on and where you left, then a modest fee collected. The drive through the big city then out to Long Island to my aunt's home was a bit scary. This was a courtesy visit and thank-you for the kindness shown me previously. We only stayed a few days as I was anxious to get on the road to British Columbia where an old uncle, Fred, my late father's elder brother, lived.

Fred Earnshaw had emigrated from Ireland in the early 1920s then homesteaded in the remote Peace River area where he, as an ex-serviceman, was granted a section, one mile by one mile, of land by the government. He made two trips back to Dublin, both financed by his parents and other relatives. At age ten I had been fascinated by his big cowboy hat and tales of life in the bush. His nearest neighbour was one-quarter mile from his shack. He, and many others, went to work in the Alberta wheat harvest in the fall and quit as soon as they had $150 saved from wages, enough to purchase flour, bacon, tea, sugar and other staples to see them through the winter. After the mean temperatures were below freezing he would shoot a buck, skin it, dress it out, then hang it up in a nearby tree with a pulley, out of reach of bears. Later he would lower it down, then with an axe chip off from the frozen carcass enough meat for a stew. His primitive log cabin was heated by a fireplace made from an oil drum on its side supported by large stones with the chimney going up through the roof. Lighting was by oil lamp; water was melted snow. We mailed him paperback novels from England to help pass the time in the long winter when days were almost dark. Talking to the chickens penned at one end of the shack and shooting pack

139

rats as they scurried around the shelves in the evenings helped to relieve the boredom. He also wrote primitive poetry which I was to read many years later.

After thirty years he had cleared about an acre from one corner of his section, enough to make a vegetable garden and accommodate the shack and root cellar. Other more industrious neighbours had wheat fields, tractors and livestock on their land and were prospering.

Our journey across the United States, staying at night in cheap boarding houses, was uneventful. Our meals were mainly cooked at the roadside on a Primus stove. The weather was fine and several side trips, including Mount Rushmore and the Badlands of South Dakota, lengthened the journey to about ten days. We presented ourselves at the Canadian Customs at Aldergrove, British Columbia. Another tedious wait ensued as we explained how June had entered the US. Then we were off to Uncle Fred's. The address was Delgany Ranch, Elk View Mountain, Sardis, BC.

In British Columbia in 1941, soon after the US entered the war against Japan, the American army was embarking on the gigantic task of putting a highway from Dawson Creek in Canada through to Alaska. Uncle Fred left his shack only a few miles away and took a job as a civilian storekeeper with the construction company. He travelled as such until the route was completed at Anchorage. He met Jane, an Irish lady who was in charge of the nursing section. The friendship blossomed into romance then finally marriage. When the job was completed Fred realized his way of life would not be acceptable to his bride. He went south to find a suitable place to live. This took him to a ninety-acre holding on Elk View Mountain, near Sardis. There was an old log cabin which pleased him plus a flock of some forty sheep which could be useful. He bought the property for $7,500, then sent for Jane. When she arrived by bus he brought her out to the property, the highest residence on the mountain with no near neighbours.

When they stepped out of the taxi she took one look and pro-nounced, 'Well if you think I'm going to live there, you're mistaken.'

Fred's reply was simple, 'Well, I am.'

Before long their few sticks of furniture arrived from the north and they moved in – with the promise that a proper house would be built as soon as possible. The shack would be relegated to store room and hen house. So it was that 'Delgany Ranch' came about. The sheep were being decimated by bears and coyotes. They no longer held their charm. Fred sold them all then bought milk goats which could be readily housed in the barn. There was a passable garden and even a horse came with the property, which helped in hauling downed trees for firewood.

It was 1954 when we drove up the mountain on a gravel road past a few homesteads then nothing for miles. We felt sure we had taken the wrong road and were looking for some place to turn around when we spotted the ranch sign and drove down a long track to the building area where we were welcomed into a pleasant house. Jane and Fred were in their late fifties. She was very Irish, tall and slim. She had travelled most of the world in her profession. They practised subsistence farming, producing almost all their living requirements: meat, milk and vegetables from the garden and goats. Jane even had a spinning wheel and produced socks, sweaters and bonnets dyed green from chlorophyll in local plants. Soap was made from the goat carcass fat plus caustic soda, a root cellar preserved most of their vegetables and their other staples were the basic flour, sugar, tea and salt.

The goat herd built up to around twenty pedigree milkers plus their young followers. The milk was picked up daily by a neighbour then sold to eager buyers in town. The meagre UK pension they both received was boosted by the Canadian Government, which passed an act providing all ex-service personnel with the more generous Canadian pensions rather than the pittance coming out from the UK. It was a great help to them.

We were nearly broke and anxiously awaited our yearly allowance from the UK which amount was rigidly controlled by export regulations. We helped with the work and got used to goat's milk, butter and cheese – and roast 'kid'. But I would soon have to find employment, and income.

CHAPTER 52

More Exams

The obvious choice was to get back into veterinary practice. I made an appointment to meet veterinary Dr Barton in the nearby town of Chilliwack then travelled with him on his farm rounds. He was a great character, very efficient in his work and humorous in his comments to the farmers, mainly in the dairy business. The day passed happily as we attended several prosperous farms, managed mostly by efficient Mennonite families. The treatment and advice on most cases was similar to my own. Around 5:00 p.m. he told me he had still to make the most important call of the day. I waited in anticipation. It was to the liquor store. From there we returned to his office where we discussed my prospects. It would be necessary for me to take a written examination to become licensed to practice. He telephoned Dr Chester, the profession's current registrar, to find out the date of the next examination and was told it would be in two days. It was after 9:00 p.m. and a nice meal served by Bernice, his wife, when I drove up the mountain to tell June we were going to Vancouver the next day. It would be a two-hour drive, our first visit to British Columbia's business metropolis.

When we arrived in the big city on the following evening I telephoned Dr Chester and told him I had recently arrived in the Province and would like to take the examination. He was most helpful and asked if I had seen any of the previous examination papers to get an idea of the type of questions. I told him I had not, adding, the only papers I was interested in seeing were the next day's, which I think shocked him. At the time, 1954, I had been qualified ten years. Surely I had forgotten most of the details of the obscure subjects in the curriculum. I presented myself at his residence along with five other hopefuls. We spent the day, with a short break for lunch, doing our best to complete the written answers. I did well on the practical questions and left the details of academia alone.

The other candidates were all recently out of college and had jobs to go to if successful. I told Dr Chester something of my veterinary background. I wanted to establish my own practice and was prepared to go where there was a need for a veterinarian. His answer buoyed my hopes.

'There's a small town in the Okanagan about one hundred fifty miles inland situated between two beautiful lakes. It has a population of about ten thousand, many of whom are in the fruit growing business. There is at present no veterinary practice but the Federal and Provincial Government vets help out where they can. There's also a local undertaker who does spays. If you go there you will have a good life – but you won't make much money.'

How right he was!

Two weeks later a telephone call informed me that I would be given the licence to practice. I had received the annual remittance from the UK. We gave Uncle Fred $300 for our board, packed all our possessions into the car, got a free road map from a local garage, and we were on our way to the city of Penticton, the next phase of my interesting career.

CHAPTER 53

The Beautiful Okanagan

The journey took most of the day through beautiful Manning Park. Soon after the entrance driving through the forested hills we came to an extensive burned area. At the roadside a large replica of a burning cigarette hung from a scaffold. Underneath a notice read, 'The person who dropped this should be hanging here.' The sign was controversial and offended some people. It was removed a few years later, long before the area became reforested. The highway was twisty and hilly and took us through picturesque scenery then the small towns of Princeton and Keremeos until finally we turned a bend and there below us was Skaha Lake. Off in the distance with glimmering lights in the gathering dusk was the city which would be our home for the next nine years. Driving down the main street we passed an open area on which sat a boarded up one-story wooden building, thirty feet back from the road. 'There,' I said to June, 'is the future Penticton Veterinary Hospital.' We found a motel then settled down for the night.

Next morning I drove out to have a closer look at the building I had spotted the previous evening. It was painted white and had a red duroid roof. The weeds around it suggested it was not inhabited. Further down on the property was a large shed. Over in a corner of the extensive grounds bordering on the road was a modern bungalow with a well-kept garden. I went over to inquire about the ownership of the property, which covered about twelve acres. The door was answered by an aged man, tall but somewhat stooped. I told him what I had in mind and he invited me in. His name was Henry Myerhoff. He had operated a circus for many years in BC. His land used to be the wintering quarters for the wagons and equipment. He had lived in the white house for many years then built the new one when he retired.

'Would you sell me the old house?' I asked.

'Well, yes,' he replied, 'but there's no land to go with it. Before we go any further don't you think you should have a look inside? Here's the key to the back door.'

Fifteen minutes later I was back then made an offer to buy it for $2,000 as long as I could have tenure for two years. That was agreed. There would also be a $7.50 charge per month for ground rent. Next I said that I would also rent the big shed for $10 a month, envisioning a kennel building for boarding dogs. That was acceptable. He suggested that I should meet him at his lawyer's office the following morning at which time we would put it all in writing. Although he abstained, he gave me a glass of wine. He seemed pleased with the deal. Before things could change I said I was a bit strapped for money and could only pay $50 a month plus the rentals.

Back at the motel, June was flabbergasted. Again I was being impatient, precipitous and foolhardy in addition to being broke. We were skimping on everything so it called for a visit to the Royal Bank where I met Roe Dinney, the manager. I told him I would like to start an account with his bank but would be operating on overdraft for some time. He said he didn't understand the term.

'Well,' I told him, 'I won't be putting anything in, just taking out, at least for a while.' He asked what my business was. When I told him he became my first client.

'Dr Earnshaw, we are going on holiday for two weeks. Do you think you could board our two cats?'

We were in. I could draw up to $1,000 a month for six months at which time my loan would be consolidated when fixed terms of repayment would be instituted. This was a major step forward. In celebration I took June to the Prince Charles Hotel for a steak dinner.

CHAPTER 54

Getting Started in Penticton

The lawyer, Frank Christian, drew up the agreement, which was duly signed. I wrote a cheque for $57.50. The shed rent would be deferred until the second month. The tenancy was to start officially on 1 August but we were welcome to take occupancy right away, which was a week early. We went to Mac and Mac, the local 'supply everything' store and arranged for credit until 1 September. We bought a bedspring and mattress which would be delivered on the following day and set up on wooden blocks. We also bought sheets and blankets, dishes, brooms and brushes plus cleaning materials. Then it was time to take my bride out to her first married home. No, I did not carry June over the threshold. She looked around, felt it was adequate, and started cleaning. There was a glassed-in porch at the front, leading into a large room that would become my consulting room, surgery, pharmacy and office. There was one bedroom, a middle room with an oil burning heater, a bathroom, a kitchen with a large coal and wood-burning stove and off this another smaller room. Happily, everything was in good repair. The water had been turned off but not disconnected. The power was still on. Apparently Meyerhoff would leave a few lights on at night to deter break-ins. We would have to get the meters changed into our name.

Finally we thought about food. June hastened over to a nearby grocery store and came back with a bag of the essentials. Next day a visit to the local second-hand store filled in the rest of the furnishings, two wooden chairs, an electric hot plate, kettle and saucepans and an old radio, all at bargain prices.

I left a note at the *Penticton Herald* newspaper where I met Grev Rowland, the owner and publisher. It was a brief item to tell the local public that Dr Earnshaw and his wife had arrived in town with the intention of opening a veterinary hospital and would welcome visits from UK ex-patriots.

Our first caller, a couple of days later, was Mrs Rowe, who was moved by the sparseness of our furnishings and returned later with two easy chairs, a lot of carpeting, and curtain material. Marion Boyd, wife of Dr David Boyd, came along and invited us to dinner, while many others dropped in to welcome the new vet and offer any help they could provide. It was very warming. In reflection it casts my thoughts back to the days when people went out of their way to help others. Happily, many still do.

Talking with the Boyds gave us a good insight into the history of the town, its commercial structure, its professional possibilities, the climate – hot as hell in summer and freezing all winter – coupled with a few suggestions which might help us get established.

The first was to go and see Dr Roy Walker, the leading medico in town, which I did on the following Monday afternoon after his last appointment. He sat behind a large desk in his office and welcomed me like a colleague. He was quite elderly, of small stature and friendly smile. He told me he was restricting the hours he now put in at the office. We chatted away and I learned what life was like in that area forty years earlier when he first came to town. Then we started talking about equipment. I told him I had nothing so far. Perhaps some of his friends had enamel dishes that were being replaced with stainless steel – the dogs wouldn't appreciate the difference. He

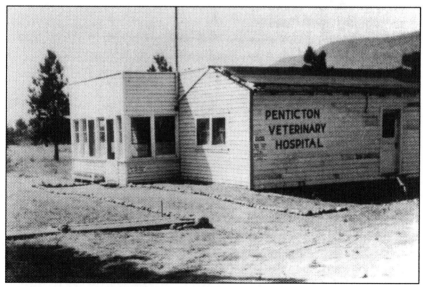

Penticton Veterinary Hospital.

suggested several things, finally saying, 'Why don't you come up to the hospital tomorrow morning at 11 o'clock when most of the doctors gather in the common room and have coffee. We'll see what we can scrounge.'

It was an excellent suggestion and garnered me deliveries of an older autoclave, numerous glass syringes with needles, lots of suture material, a variety of forceps and scalpels and, most important, an introduction to a wonderful group of professionals, many of whom became friends and clients. The radiologist told me if I ever needed an X-ray of an animal there was a handy back way into his department. It proved invaluable.

I compiled a list of further things I needed then phoned the office of Pitman-Moore, an office supply company in Vancouver, who were more than willing to extend credit to a new establishment. A few more furnishings, erecting some shelving, cutting the weeds, a minor roof repair, then when my drug supplies arrived I was ready to open. Finally, a paint job on the building was done by a local firm. We went out for the day, returning as the work was nearly completed. Large letters of black paint on the side of the building announced to the public: 'Penticton Vetinry Hospital.' It was corrected the following day. We were in business.

CHAPTER 55

Rumen 'Windows'

It wasn't long after the telephone was installed that the small animal side of the practice became busy. I decided to have office hours in the afternoon and evening, leaving the mornings for surgery – spays and other cases needing an anaesthetic. Ranch calls were not frequent as beef cattle were out on the range during summer and fall. When off colour in yards during the winter they were often doctored by their owners who had always done so with ready access to antibiotics, and knew how to give them. There were no dairy herds except at the Summerland Research Station where about twenty-five Jerseys were maintained for experimental purposes.

Jim Miltimore was doing work on bloat which occurs when cattle are put out on rapidly growing spring pasture, especially if rich in clover. After eating too much of it the rapid fermentation and formation of gas seemed to make it difficult to belch, causing the rumen to fill up with gas, sometimes to such a degree that pressure on the diaphragm would cause respiratory distress and even death. The normal treatment is to give a medication by mouth to stop the fermentation. In more serious cases, one could push a sharpened metal tube through the skin, muscle and wall of the rumen to relieve the pressure of the gasses – which, incidentally, are highly flammable should you be lighting a cigarette. To go more deeply into the analysis and chemistry of the process Jim consulted me on the possibility of inserting a perspex 'window' with a screw-on lid into the rumen. This would allow access to the contents so that samples could be taken before and after the 'bloat', the whole process being timed. Also various antibloat medications could be tested.

'You make 'em and I'll put 'em in,' I told him – and so four of his cows got the windows, which assisted him in his experiments.

There was no bull at the farm and the transportation of freshly calved cows from the government farm at Agassiz was a nuisance so artificial insemination using frozen semen was adopted and required me to make two or three visits a week as there were several repeats.

Traumatic reticulitis was a problem. This condition occurs in the second stomach when a piece of metal, often wire, penetrates the wall anteriorly, causing inflammation and pain. Depending on the length of the wire or nail, it sometimes reaches the heart membranes and can be fatal. The bits of wire are common where wire is used in the hay baling process and some bits of it are left around to be consumed when the field is subsequently grazed or in the hay itself. The symptoms are 'painful indigestion'. I wrote to Dr McLintock in England for a rubber sleeve he had perfected for use in the operation to remove the offending foreign body, which minimized contamination of the tissues by stomach contents. I used it successfully several times and also demonstrated its use at the annual convention of the BC Veterinary Association. When magnets became available to be given the cows by mouth they clumped any metallic objects together which then lay harmlessly in the bottom of the reticulum – a brilliant idea.

Fees were a problem. The two government vets had charged very little for vaccination and spaying of cats and dogs. When I started the practice I asked both to desist but their co-operation was tardy and later on I had to be more forceful. Distemper vaccinations cost $9, spays were $25 and my consulting fee $10 but often paid under protest. For a while the bank was keeping us.

CHAPTER 56

Hunting the Blue Grouse

Penticton is a lovely city, nestled between two large lakes with hills on either side. It is about two miles long and one mile wide. It has a long Main Street with secondary roads running parallel. When I was there the business area was confined to the north end while numerous motels dotted the southern end. Nowadays huge shopping malls extend throughout, it being the business centre for a wide area. The residential development spread out on both sides. It has become a tourist mecca during the summer months when families enjoy the sandy beaches and ready supply of fruit from the orchards, which was the principal industry. In winter Apex ski resort attracts many enthusiasts. When I was there the railroad from the Kootenays passed through to Vancouver. My nearest veterinary neighbours were thirty-five miles to the north and one hundred and fifty miles to the west, with nobody to the south and east, it being thirty miles to the US border and one hundred and thirty-five miles to the Alberta border.

One of my early clients was Major Hugh Fraser, who lived at Okanagan Falls. He was of British extraction, claiming relationship to a famous naval Admiral of the same name. He kept beautiful collies as pets. He lived in a fine house on a hillside above Vasseau Lake which he named S.Y.L. ranch. The initials spelled 'See You Later'. I was told he had been married many years ago to a lady who had come from England. She detested both the freezing winters and boiling summers and left the place after less than a year. He also owned a working ranch a few miles away at Okanagan Falls managed by Russell Spears who tended some horses and a few beef cows. I asked the Major if I could go to the ranch, which bordered on the government-owned hills, to do some shooting. He readily agreed and gave me Russell's telephone number.

It was our first October in the Okanagan. Russell suggested we go after the blue grouse which live mainly at the higher elevations feeding on the bountiful supply of berries in the fall. He asked me to come down to the ranch one Sunday with a packed lunch where he would have horses ready at 10:00 a.m. On a clear, sunny morning Russell and I set off for the hills. He was a grizzled individual about fifty, dressed cowboy fashion with jeans, chaps, leather jacket and Stetson hat. He was not very talkative. This was my first experience of a western saddle, which I found quite comfortable. I had borrowed a double-barrelled 20-gauge shotgun, more than adequate for any bird up to forty yards but requiring a greater degree of accuracy than the larger 12-bore. Up through the woods we rode. The area was not heavily treed and allowed views of picturesque Skaha Lake from our vantage point. When we reached the higher elevations there was a flutter of wings as five or more 'blues' took flight from the sparse cover and alighted in a tall fir tree about fifty yards away. We both dismounted and tied the horses to nearby trees. Then we crept slowly forward with guns ready. When we were about forty yards from the fir tree I could see several birds sitting on the upper branches. I stood up and said, 'OK, Russell, flush them.'

He rapidly replied, 'You silly bugger, if you don't shoot now you won't get any.'

My sportsmanship demanded that you didn't shoot a sitting bird. I had a lot to learn. We shot several using similar tactics. I only got one 'on the wing' and was surprised at the speed of their take-off. I came home with four birds and prepared them for the table a few days later by removing the plump breasts and putting them in a roasting pan with a strip of bacon over each, some chopped onion, seasoning and four peeled potatoes. This was to be our first dinner for guests. The Boyds were invited to our humble abode where our cutlery was primitive, our wine glasses tumblers, the table a four-seater. The kitchen stove was fired up with wood and, apart from almost putting us out of the house with the heat, produced an excellent meal.

Russell and I made several forays into the hills, each time taking birds home for the pot. The snows would soon be coming and would bring the deer down from the high places. Then we would hunt for venison.

CHAPTER 57

Deer Hunts

Snows appeared on the surrounding hills. Winter was fast approaching. Our oil barrel was topped up to fuel the space heater and we bought warm clothing. A carpenter had built several dog cages for the expected boarders and a six-foot high wooden fence was erected around the shed to provide an exercise yard. A double entrance to prevent any escapes was built where the outer door was closed before the inner one was opened. Cats were housed within our abode, the original boxes with chicken wire being replaced with some far better, purchased from the pet store. The house was well insulated. Doors and windows fitted snugly to eliminate drafts. We equipped the Ford with snow tires to prepare for the expected ranch calls – which were slow in coming. Snow at the lower level entailed daily sweeping a pathway to the front door and down to the kennel building, now also equipped with an oil-burning heater which had to be fuelled up every third day. A nuisance but it made the doggies comfortable and impressed the owners who were making that side of the business quite profitable. June and I were doing all the chores – and enjoying it.

Russell phoned to say he wanted to get his winter's supply of deer meat. Could I go down to Okanagan Falls on the following Sunday? I was keen. I bought an old army Lee Enfield 303 in which the stock had been trimmed to look like a sporting rifle. On horseback we set off soon after 9:00 a.m., well wrapped up. It was snowing lightly as we made our way to the higher elevations. We saw only a few deer tracks. Around noon Russell suggested that we split up and meet later at the double pine, an anomaly which we had seen previously several times. I was doubtful that I could find the meeting place but agreed reluctantly. The estimated time to get there was 1:30 p.m. If I needed help or shot a deer I was to fire three shots in rapid succession then he would come to my assistance.

About an hour later as I rode higher up the hills I spotted four or five mule deer some one hundred yards ahead on a rise. I quickly

153

dismounted, tied the horse to a young fir tree, and doffed my heavy jacket, which I hung on the saddle. Taking only the rifle, I crept carefully forward. The deer had disappeared when I got up the rise. I saw them again moving slowly over the next rise. I needed to have a still shot. I followed them for probably fifteen minutes but each time I spotted them they were moving ahead. Then I never saw them again. I scouted around for a while then gave up the hunt. Now I had to find my horse. I must confess to being very much a novice in the woods and probably did all the wrong things. I couldn't find Dobbin. I whinnied, hoping to hear a reply but it was the wrong whinney. Now I had to take stock of things. I fired three times which Russell apparently did not hear. He had shot a large buck and was busy gutting it. I was some five miles 'up the hill' in shirtsleeves and fully six inches of snow. I would have to move quickly if I was to reach the ranch before darkness. It was a hectic journey, climbing over downed trees, sliding down gullies then panting up others. I was sweating profusely. As the light was fading I reached the barbed wire fence that surrounded the ranch pastures.

Russell was home and had a meal ready. I would have to come down early the next morning when we would go up to rescue the horse and get the deer he had shot, which would by then be frozen. This time we set out at daybreak. When we reached the outside of the fence we heard a whinney and there was Dobbin standing placidly. My jacket still hung from the saddle. By good fortune I had tied him to a sapling from which he had managed to pull free. Russell took my horse while I took Dobbin back to the ranch, took off the saddle and gave him a rub down. I put a blanket over him and fed him some oats and hay. Then I went back to work.

My next deer hunt was more successful. Walt Cousins was the by-law officer for the city. He belonged to the Fish and Game Club which had over a hundred members. They were very active in promoting range shoots and fishing derbies. Walt suggested we go to a place he knew in Summerland. It was on a hill overlooking the lake where the deer would go for a drink during the night and wend their way up the hill in the first light of dawn. We would be waiting for them. I spotted a doe on her way up. If I kept quiet and hidden she would pass quite near to me. I shot her at a range of only twenty yards. Then remorse and regret set in. Walt came over and we loaded the carcass into the trunk of his car.

'Walt,' I said, 'that's both the first and the last deer I'm ever going to shoot. I don't want any of it.' A few weeks later we went to his house for dinner – and were both a bit squeamish when deer steaks were the main course.

CHAPTER 58

Brucellosis Vaccination

In September I received a letter from the Veterinary Department of the Provincial Government asking if I would undertake the brucellosis vaccination of all heifers aged between six and nine months in my practice area. These would have been born on the range in spring then in the fall brought to the vicinity of the ranch where they would be fed hay during the winter. At this time the young males are castrated and all are branded with the particular identification of the owner's ranch. The payment for vaccination was $1.00 for each one injected then ear-tagged. All materials were provided. I jumped at the chance and contacted the various ranchers' organizations in my area. The work would commence in late November.

The Princeton ranches were to be first. I loaded up vaccine and ear-tags and an overnight bag for what was estimated to be a two-day job. After a forty-mile drive on a frosty morning, I booked into the only hotel and was met by a young rancher named Trehearn. He was to accompany me to the various ranches, where it was hoped the young heifers would have been segregated from the steers and could be run through the chute then, when packed together, be given the vaccine somewhere in the neck. I had a repeater syringe holding ten five-ml doses. It took longer to load up than to dispense the contents after which a metal numbered tag was clipped into the right ear. Most ranchers were co-operative and had the heifers ready. By 4:30 p.m. we had vaccinated more than three hundred, a good day's work. It was dark at this time so it surprised me to learn that there was more to come. Trehearn told me we had to go up into the hills for eighteen miles to Missoula Lake where Bill Shopshire had a small spread. The narrow snow-covered gravel road led through a forest. I was told, 'If a logging truck comes down you must get off the road as they can't stop on this slippery surface.' Fortunately, none came at any time I went up there.

Bill, a rugged individual, welcomed us with a big smile – and a hot rum for which we were grateful. He had sent his wife and two children into town for winter schooling while he 'batched' at the ranch. When the rum had disappeared he produced a fine dinner of beef stew which was the first good meal since breakfast. It was fully nine o'clock when a move was made to do the work. I had brought my stuff into the house to prevent freezing and divested all the outer clothing in the warm kitchen. Now I put it on again to venture into the frosty night. It was ten degrees below freezing. Some twenty young Herefords milled around in the corral, steers and heifers together. Bill produced a lariat and by moonlight lassoed a heifer, which was then snubbed up to a central post, steadied by Treahern and vaccinated and tagged by me. In this way eleven heifers were injected when Bill announced, 'That's all.' It was an amazing performance. We'd had a great evening with a really incredible man.

As we left I thanked Bill for his hospitality, adding, 'Next time I'll bring the rum.' We all laughed.

On the drive back to the hotel Trehearn told me, he, like a number of other young ranchers, had married a school teacher who had been sent into the area. They had three young children. It was past midnight when I dropped him by his car near the hotel. We shook hands and he said he had enjoyed the day and Will Brown would be at the hotel at 9:00 a.m. to guide me on the second day. Then he added, 'Oh, did I tell you, Bill Shopshire is blind in one eye.'

CHAPTER 59

Perils of Winter

Ray Green was a friendly old timer who ranched half way up Green Mountain, named after one of his pioneer ancestors. He was a cripple, bent almost double. I never really learned why. However, I did see on his living room wall a photograph of a strapping young cowboy dressed up with a white Stetson, jeans and chaps. He said to me as I washed my hands in the sink, 'That's me as a young 'un.' I had previously been up to the ranch to treat an old horse which was losing condition and not eating well. After filing the sharp points off the molar teeth with the tooth float I recommended it be fed half a bucket of boiled barley daily with some salt added in addition to its usual fare until the horse was fleshed in a bit more to his liking. It solved the problem.

One cold, miserable morning a week before Christmas I went up there to vaccinate twenty-five young heifers for brucellosis. I had to navigate a snow covered road for about a mile and a half, with frequent bends and switchbacks as it wound around the mountain gaining height. Ray greeted me, apologizing for the inclement weather and the temperature, which at 10:00 a.m. was eleven degrees below freezing. I left the car engine running with the vaccine in the warmth until needed. Ray had two seasoned cowboys to help run the heifers into the chute where I administered the 'shot'. They should have been done in half an hour but these heifers were wild and continually broke away when being herded in the corral by his not too nimble helpers. I stood around for long spells and got progressively more chilled. It annoyed me because I had arranged to visit another ranch for a similar job on the same morning. Ted Stuart wouldn't be happy to have his cowboys and heifers waiting around. When we finished the vaccinations Ray went into the house. A minute later he came out with a twenty-six-ounce bottle of Scotch whisky which was opened and passed around the four of us. It was very welcome and sent a surge of warmth and comfort through me. When it came around a second time I hesitated, but the inner warm glow suggested a further swallow – or two – and soon the bottle was empty.

I thanked Ray and his helpers, climbed into my sturdy station wagon and headed down the mountain's icy road. Before long I realized I was travelling too fast. I geared down but didn't dare do any more than touch very briefly on the brake pedal. At each curve I slithered all over the place. The awful realization that I might soon flip completely off the roadway dawned. It was not a comforting thought. More by chance than skill I hit the final curve still going about forty miles an hour. This time I could not hold the car. It went off the icy road, bouncing along the sturdy barbed wire fence of the Stuart ranch with a ripping and tearing noise for some forty yards. The front wheel hit a large rock which bounced the car back onto the road again. I was shaking but in one piece.

I drove into the Stuart place and up to the ranch house, got out and went inside. I was flushed and shaky and thickened in speech as I asked Stuart to go outside and check the far side of my station wagon, which had skidded off the road and possibly demolished his fence. He reported all the damage was superficial which a body shop could easily repair, and not to worry about the fence. They never alluded to my condition, which was drunkenness. And they will never know unless they read this book. But I still wonder.

CHAPTER 60

We Buy a House

By the end of our first winter we were confident the practice would be a success and afford us a reasonable income. Currency regulations in Britain were being relaxed and it was now possible to export money. We went to the bank, thanked them for their assistance in getting us established, and opened a regular chequeing account. We also began looking for better accommodation. The real estate firm of A.F. Cumming was very helpful. The owner, Archie Cumming, told us the old 'bank house' was for sale for $6500. It had not been advertised thus far. He would be very pleased to show it, a two-story house located on the prestigious 'Middle Bench', the higher land to the east of the city. It had a quarter of an acre of well-manicured grounds with a detached garage, shade and fruit trees, lawns and a grapevine. At first sight we fell in love and told Archie we would buy the house if he could arrange a modest down payment. 'Well let's talk about it over a cup of tea,' he replied. 'You see, I live next door.'

Some time later he told me that, rather than advertise it generally, he personally met all prospective buyers to ensure compatible neighbours.

It was no problem to find a retired single man to live in the hospital building and take care of the janitorial duties and feed the boarding dogs. June furnished the house very tastefully and we entered the Penticton social whirl of dinner parties, barbecues, card games and general entertaining. Relatives came to visit from the UK and two female cousins stayed through a summer, working in the fruit packing houses.

Life went on very pleasantly. I negotiated with the City Council to purchase land in the light industrial area and bought one and a half acres as a site for my new hospital which was built and functioning just two years after our arrival. The old building was sold to the yacht club for one dollar. A major transportation project began to jack it up, put it on a low-bed truck and bring it through

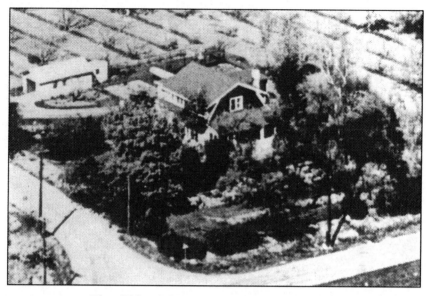

The old bank house, our home for nine years.

the main street at 2:00 p.m. on a Saturday afternoon. All the work was done by volunteers, mainly West Coast Transmission and Canadian Pacific Railway personnel. The journey, particularly along the narrow roadway at the water's edge on the south shore of Okanagan Lake, was precarious. We nearly lost the whole building in getting it to the new location. Under the supervision of several experts it came to rest partly over the water on piles which had been driven earlier. It was the Penticton Yacht Club's premises for many years. A well-stocked bar supervised by Ira Johnson became a lunchtime venue for beer and a sandwich. In the evenings it often attracted gamblers and philosophers who had little inclination to spend their time at home. A large deck was built over the water where we held dances on Saturday evenings during the summer months. They were very happy, well attended affairs. The coloured lights plus clear skies and moored boats enhanced the general ambience.

The clean ups on Sunday mornings had their moments. On one occasion much of the decorative fish net had fallen into the water and now held six large carp flopping around in the mesh. John Glass later took them down to the Chinese restaurant on Front Street where Manny Lee rubbed his hands, contemplating an abundant

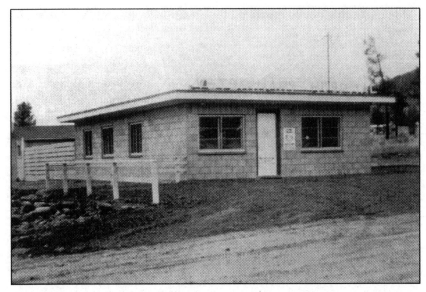

The new Penticton Veterinary Hospital.

supply for his seafood specials. John was invited to bring his family in for a free dinner.

The practice was a tie. Not until old Dr Dunbar, a retired veterinarian from the prairies, came to town did I think of a holiday in the UK. He did not know much about small animal practice but agreed to take care of things if we were away for a month. And so after four years absence we went to England to enjoy meeting up with family and old friends, with whom I had kept in touch through our annual Christmas letters. June was 'expecting'. When it came time to return, her doctor mistakenly told her she was further advanced than she thought. It would not be advisable to travel, at that time, by sea. I came home alone. Four months later she arrived back with a baby boy.

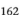

CHAPTER 61

Robbie Roberts

I first met Robbie Roberts when he was appointed the SPCA inspector for Penticton. This position had been under discussion at executive meetings for several weeks when his credentials were debated. He was forty-five years old. He had been born at Peachland, a small community further up the lake, where his father had a string of saddle horses for hire to holiday tourists, an industry that was then in its infancy. Robbie had served in the Provost Corps of the Canadian Army during the war with postings mainly in the UK from where he had returned with an English bride.

Growing up in an area such as Peachland on the shores of Okanagan Lake with a hinterland of rolling forested hills must have been a wonderful experience for Robbie. The fishing, in both the lake and streams, was excellent. In addition to the horses Roberts senior had the Government contract to refuel the oil burning navigation light on Rattlesnake Island, some two miles away on the opposite side of the lake. He had fashioned primitive fishing lures using a five-inch length of stick with a screw ring at the rounded front end while a triple hook was spliced into the tapered rear end. When splashed with different coloured paints it became a fishing lure. He towed a couple of these behind the boat whenever he rowed across the lake, which was every fourth day, catching one or two eight- to ten-pound salmon on most trips.

Grouse and deer were plentiful with no restrictions on bag limits. When Robbie was in his early teens he was allowed to lead the string of horses which took groups of fishermen or hunters back into the hills. The average group of hunters was three or four, mostly men, usually from the US or Europe. Camping equipment, food, and supplies were carried on packhorses.

On one occasion the group was traversing a sloping area of shale. Robbie asked the hunters to dismount then lead their horses across the hazardous area. One large fellow riding a mare whose three-month-old foal was travelling with her paid no attention. Robbie walked back, took hold of the bridle to steady the mare, then glared up at the big American. 'Get down off your horse, you son of a bitch or I will drag you off,' he admonished. The rider dismounted with a smile on his face.

Later in the evening when they sat around the campfire one of the hunters took Robbie aside to confide in him. 'That fellow on the mare this morning is Gene Tunney, the ex-world heavyweight boxing champion.'

Incidentally, as the floatplane taking this party back to the States from Penticton was taxiing for take off the wing of the plane hit the wharf. The passengers were rescued then continued their homeward journey by bus.

In addition to taking care of the pound animals Inspector Roberts' duties included catching stray dogs or cats then housing them for a limited time, after which they would be sold or put down. He also picked up dogs that had been hit on the highway by incautious motorists.

I loaned Robbie my captive bolt pistol so that he could dispatch his indigents in a proper manner. We met often as I referred clients to him when they needed transportation for sick animals. He did his job well, investigating several complaints of animal cruelty in a wide area. In those where he felt a prosecution was warranted I was called as an expert witness. Most of the cases occurred in late winter when feed supplies had been used up and cattle or horses were becoming emaciated.

The law at that time could do little to convict on the charge of cruelty to animals because the written charge included the word 'wilful'. It had to be shown that the rancher or horse owner had wilfully set out to starve his animals, which was far from the case and impossible to prove.

One morning Robbie brought to the hospital a dead deer which had been killed on the road bordering the lake north of the city. It was emaciated or starved. This is confirmed by cracking open a long bone of the leg where the marrow shows as a watery fluid instead of the fat-laden marrow. I telephoned the Game Warden, Butch Tyler, whom I had met, to alert him to a situation decimating the deer population in the area. It was my hope that bales of hay could be scattered in the area to sustain the starving deer for a few weeks until the spring arrived with its forage bounty. Butch was not pleased when I told him the local paper would be asked to alert the public to this sad situation.

'First of all,' he said, 'I am going to charge you with being in possession of a deer carcass while out of season.'

I told him I would welcome that because it would bring the matter to wider public attention after it was reported in the Provincial press. He calmed down then and told me this was an annual happening after a long winter where snows covered the hills and there was little for the deer to eat.

I have learned since that a wire fence has been built there along an extensive distance to prevent deer crossing the highway.

CHAPTER 62

Moose Hunt

Robbie Roberts and I got along very well. He enjoyed company and much to the chagrin of the SPCA committee who paid his wages he found it mostly in the bar of the Canadian Legion. After his duties at the pound including feeding the normally five or six stray or lost dogs he made a cursory drive around the town but by 11 a.m. one knew where to find him.

His wife Wynn was the last to learn of this or maybe did not want to. When telephone calls came in of an urgent nature she relayed them to my office which we then passed on to Rob. The problem was not solvable. Threats of dismissal fell on deaf ears.

One day he came to see me then asked if I would give him a written testimonial relating to his present employment, his character and suitability for employment.

'What's in the wind then, Rob?' I asked.

'Well,' he replied, 'Wynn has always wanted to go back to England where all her family live and where she was far happier. I am going to apply for a job as inspector with the British RSPCA.'

I would be happy to, Rob,' I replied,' though I will miss you. Is there no alternative?'

His mind was made up. Three weeks later he told me he had been offered a job and would be leaving in about six weeks. It was the third week in September. 'Doc,' he said, 'there's one thing I would like to do before we go. Would you join me on a moose hunt in Wells Grey Park for a few days after the 1st of October when the hunting season opens?'

My feelings towards killing deer were negative, possibly because my first – and last – kill was a beautiful doe. Maybe a beast as big as a bull would be different. But friendship for Rob overcame any negative thoughts and we set about making our plans.

Wells Grey Park is in a remote area some 150 miles further north. In area it would be comparable to that of a British county like Hampshire. Within the confines of the park were mountainous heights, thick forests, grassy plains and several lakes, the largest of which was twenty miles long. I learned a lot about the project from Doug Younghusband who was the herdsman at the Summerland Experimental station. He hunted in the same area for his winter meat, usually successfully. He advised that we estimated our food needs for four days and instructed our wives to prepare this. Then we should get hold of a tent from the local Scout group with mattresses, a couple of down sleeping bags, sight our rifles in .303 or 30-30, quite acceptable, and pack plenty of cigarettes. We should take a boat packed with all we would need then travel up the lake to get away from the parking area at the south end where most of the hunters parked their cars and went forth on foot.

My sail boat would suit. It was 18ft. long, very light and presently rested in my garden on its trailer with its mast taken down and covered with a tarpaulin. It was ideal.

All we needed was a sturdy piece of board screwed on to the transom to mount a 7.5 h.p. outboard motor which I was able to borrow from Bob Gordon.

On a Tuesday evening about 7 p.m., when it was still quite light, we set off in my station wagon towing the heavily laden and well covered boat. Some fifteen miles further up the highway on the shores of Okanagan Lake we came to Peachland, a small village which had been Robbie's home as a youth. Well, we couldn't pass the Peachland Hotel bar. Maybe some of his old pals were there. An hour and two pints later we went on to Kelowna across the lake bridge then to the Capri Hotel pub . . . to see who was there. Robbie didn't know anybody but was soon in deep conversation with a small group about our hunting prospects.

Then it was closing time and another two pints later. We headed north to the city of Vernon where we arrived about midnight. There was only one possible place to go and that was the Legion. After directions from a sparse pedestrian population we found it with its bar open and ten or more patrons. Strangely, Robbie was welcomed by several who knew him from Penticton association. He livened up the place, involving the company in a competition where a matchstick was balanced on the edge of the bar. Each contestant was positioned two paces from the bar, then he had to cover one eye with the left hand, take one pace forward and with the middle finger of the right hand attempt to swipe the match off the bar with one downward stroke. After several attempts I don't think anyone made it the first time, which indicated the inebriated state of the late night revellers. It was fun and engendered a lot of laughter, ribald comments and ignoring of the barman who called 'Time gentlemen please' repeatedly.

We were both illegal and oblivious. We staggered out about 1:30 a.m., this time only three glasses worse off but still able to navigate, barely.

Next we had to find the way to Kamloops where we would turn north. Robbie was fortunate in being able to fall into a deep sleep punctuated with resonant snores which reminded me that I was helping Rob to enjoy a farewell fling in the country where he had grown up, enjoyed life, and maybe would never see again.

We had over a hundred miles to drive in the middle of the night. It was 5 a.m. when I pulled up outside the the Clearwater Hotel which was the jumping off place for the gravel road that would take us to the park. I was able to doze until being finally wakened by other traffic moving about. It was 7:15 a.m. The coffee shop should be open. After a good breakfast we found the local provision store and bought our final supplies – bread, milk, eggs and bacon.

We fuelled up then set out on the thirty-five mile drive to the lake through sparsely populated farming areas, dense forests, bridges over deep canyons and little traffic. By noon we reached the cleared area at the south end of the lake, launched the boat, parked and locked the car and took off on a clear cool afternoon with no wind and high hopes. The trip was uneventful as I persuaded Rob that it was his turn at navigation while I enjoyed a good sleep. He woke me around five o'clock as he turned into the shore where a clearing suggested a camp site. We pulled the boat up the shore and unloaded our gear, put up the tent and scouted round for firewood. There were several downed trees not far away and the bucking saw we had brought along soon had sawn a good pile of dried wood for our cooking and night time fire.

We still had an hour of daylight so I suggested we went fishing. We had lots of tackle for the light rods but unfortunately had left the can of succulent worms (three days digging in my garden) in the car. It didn't make much difference. We fished where a stream entered the lake, casting little red spinners twenty yards from the boat then bringing a two pound rainbow trout in with almost every second cast. When we had six we returned to camp and gutted them all. We left four down by the water on the sand which seemed the coolest place. After stoking up the fire I prepared a grilled trout meal which was the first since breakfast accompanied by buttered crusty bread rolls.

Afterwards we sat by the fire, Robbie chain smoking, as I listened to his exploits of growing up, through a wild adolescence, being in the Provost Corps of the Canadian Army during the war in Europe in 1944 and afterwards. His love of motor bikes and exuberant nature brought him to membership of the 'ton up club' – being clocked at 100 m.p.h., and the acid test which was crossing the London-Brighton road at sixty miles an hour when Sunday morning traffic was at its heaviest. When Rob had brought Wynn, a war bride, out to Canada they landed in Halifax which was the cheapest fare, then set off for Penticton on a motorbike and sidecar, Wynn in the sidecar with all their worldly possessions, in early winter. It was nearly 2,600 miles. The only puncture occurred when they were seven miles from their destination.

It had been a long day. Both sleepy, we resolved to be up at 7 a.m. for the first hunt, then hit the sack.

When I woke up after a lengthy and deep sleep Rob was nowhere to be found. I dressed, lit the fire and prepared a bacon and eggs breakfast for his return. But time went by and at 9 o'clock I ate heartily in spite of singed hands after manipulating the frying pan and toast over a well fuelled fire. Incidentally we had brought a can of kerosene which always ensured a good start to combustion.

A tired Robbie strolled in around ten fifteen. He had made a wide circle from our camp, climbing over felled trees and sloshing through swampy areas, but seeing no sign of Mr Moose. When he came back from the lakeshore after filling the kettle he asked me what I had done with the fish. 'Ain't seen them,' I told him. When we later went down to the shore we noticed multiple tracks of a small animal which Rob told me would have been a wolverine. It had apparently found a laid-on supper.

We sat around chatting, replenished our firewood supply and gazed across the calm lake where in the distance snow-covered mountains towered to five thousand feet or more. We were at peace with the world, not having brought a radio. Looking down the lake we were attracted to something swimming in the water. Rob fished out the binoculars then exclaimed, 'Doc, there's a moose swimming across the lake only half a mile away.' Unfortunately it was going to the opposite shore. But we now knew there were some around.

Later in the afternoon we launched the boat and went fishing again, this time coming back with a dozen nice trout which were gutted then hung up in a tree out of harm's way – or so we hoped.

Next morning was a repetition of the first. I begged off the hunt and attended to my culinary duties. Robbie arrived back after a couple of hours still with a negative report, and more exhausted the ever. After a meal we decided to go up the Azure River and into Azure Lake where there would be comparable fishing. I had learned from Doug that after heading into the river at the north end of the lake we would find quite a strong current of about 5 knots. At best my outboard could push us along at 6¹/₂ knots. It would be a slow trip. Further I had to remember to hug the right bank for two hundred yards, then come over to the left side for the next half mile. After that it should be plain sailing for another half mile to the entrance of Azure Lake, a reportedly picturesque setting.

It was nip and tuck to get ahead but after probably half an hour I estimated that we had advanced two hundred yards and headed across the twenty yards to the left bank. But we were still over shallow water and suddenly we were not moving forward but being swept down the river broadside. Yes, we had sheared a pin stabilising the propeller. It took but a few minutes and we were in the lake. We pulled in to the side and put in a spare pin and started out again. This time we made it. We enjoyed more excellent fishing and came back to camp in the late afternoon with a couple of dozen nice trout.

Our camp site was being raided by large black birds which we found were ravens. Our trout hung over a tree branch which though well out of reach of wolverine was now the dining venue for the local scavengers. Our new catch was wrapped in plastic sheets and put in the tent. I learned later that food should never be kept inside the sleeping tent as it would attract marauding grizzlies, maybe during the night.

Next day I got up early with Rob and took him in the boat to the other side of the lake about half a mile away and said I would come back in three hours to pick up him and his moose. But it wasn't to be. He had seen a moose and trailed it for an hour only to hear a shot from another hunter and come upon the dead bull moose being butchered by three others. They offered him to take all the meat he wanted but he declined.

Back at camp he was quite depressed and took himself off to have a quiet smoke while I lit the fire. He came rushing back.

'Doc, there's a caribou swimming across the lake heading straight for the camp. Where the hell are the binoculars?' ... but he had found them and was already focussing while I searched for my rifle. It turned out to be a boat with a caribou rack (antlers) fixed on the front. Two hunters arrived soon after. Their first words were, 'Got any cigarettes?' Rob was able to supply them.

Both were middle aged, growing beards after two weeks in the bush. They had set out for a trophy caribou. The herd made an annual migration through the park across a mountain pass at two thousand feet.

The hunters had made camp at a lower level then trekked up the mountainside daily but had seen nothing in the expected area. In desperation they decided to stay up the mountain overnight in order to be there at dawn. The temperature went down to 15 degrees below freezing while they sat under the trees wrapped in multiple blankets. The sound of pounding hooves and bellows of the bulls awakened them in dawn's early light when they beheld the passage of several hundred caribou on their way to a distant calving reserve. They were able to pick out a magnificent bull with a well developed rack which they shot.

Next came the chore of sawing off the rack and parts of the hind quarters. Most hunters in similar circumstances are already encumbered with much heavy gear and only take a limited amount of meat. The rack and about fifteen pounds of meat was all each could carry. The rest was left for the bears, wolves and scavengers.

One of them who had viewed the fire, and empty frying pan went to their boat and came came back with four caribou steaks which I was happy to cook. After a good meal and some more cigarettes from Rob they went on their way.

The failure of a hunt is always an anticlimax. Though Rob tried to put on a good front it was nevertheless a disappointment.

On Sunday morning we packed up all our gear and headed home.

We shared the fish and were told by both Wynn and June that they were glad not to have to wrestle with moose stew. I had enjoyed the outing, wonderful scenery and good company. Rob didn't say much.

Several years later as I sat in an English pub with Rob who was wearing his RSPCA inspector's uniform he turned to me and said, 'You know, Doc, if we had crossed the lake fifteen minutes earlier I would have bagged that moose.'

CHAPTER 63

Caesarian Section – and Dr Green

On Sundays we managed to get away for a while. Other vets practising in the Okanagan Valley were Paddy Clerke at Kelowna, about thirty-five miles further north, Lee Parkhill at Vernon, another thirty and Rod Sylvester fifteen further on. We decided to have monthly meetings during the summer to discuss mutual problems – such as low fees. At one get-together I described a condition I had seen where several spayed bitches two or three years old developed what I called para lumbar abscesses. In all cases opening and cleaning then inserting a seaton to provide drainage effected a complete cure. The cause eluded me. I sent samples of the abscess contents down to the Government Laboratory to determine the bacterial content and started to write a complete case history for submission to our veterinary journal. While doing so another case came in. Under general anaesthetic I opened the abscess and carefully removed the contents. Surprise, surprise – I found a piece of knotted silk. A thorough questioning of the owner revealed that the bitch had been spayed two years previously by the local undertaker. The wrong ligature material had been used to tie off the ovarian blood vessels which had ultimately been rejected by the body. I had been saved an embarrassing situation should I have rushed into print.

It was early spring when Paddy Clerke phoned around lunchtime. 'Ernie,' he asked, 'have you ever done a caesarian section on a mare?'

'Done several,' I lied.

He then went on to describe a situation where he had attended a mare belonging to a local doctor. It was a foaling case. Only the head of the foal had passed through the vaginal passage to the exterior. There was virtually no room for Paddy to get his arm in and bring up the legs owing to the mare being excessively fat. He had tried for some time but had given up. The foal was dead. It was either a major surgical operation or shoot the mare. I said, 'Paddy, get some instruments sterilized, plenty of help and be prepared to give the anaesthetic. I will be at your hospital at 2:00 p.m. Have the mare trucked in to your place.'

As I drove to Kelowna I realized this would be a major undertaking as very few such operations had been done successfully. Looking back I am surprised at my courage.

The mare was anaesthetised using chloral hydrate solution intravenously, rolled on to her back, legs tied down, and supported there with bales of straw. The abdomen was clipped of hair, scrubbed, then soaked with iodine. Towels were affixed with clips to avoid any contamination. We were left with a midline operation site two feet long and one wide. The surgery went well. After making a bold incision into the abdomen the uterus was brought up, incised for eighteen inches then, after removing the foal's head, the rest of the body was 'exteriorized'. Then followed a lengthy suturing job using strong catgut to repair the tissues then tape on the skin. The operation had taken over two hours. The mare got to her feet with lots of help and was prevented from falling by the several hands who assisted her to the nearest loose box in Paddy's yard. Large doses of penicillin were to follow for several days.

I kept in touch with Paddy by phone each day. The reports were not good. The mare looked very poorly, had not eaten and had a 'tucked up' appearance. Prospects were bad. On the third day after the operation Paddy told me the doctor felt she should be put down.

'Not after all that trouble,' I told him. 'She hasn't run a temperature so there's probably no infection. All we have to do is get her to eat or give her water and nourishment by stomach tube. There is another way, Paddy: search around until you find some fresh new grass and offer it.'

That evening Paddy was jubilant on the phone. 'The mare has eaten the grass and perked up.' It was a major turning point. 'Dr Green' had done it again.

CHAPTER 64

A. Dunbar, DVM

Old Doc Dunbar, whom I have mentioned in a previous chapter, came to Penticton to retire after a long and sometimes successful veterinary career on the prairies. Tall and in good fettle, he had a kindly face. Although somewhat portly he was active and regularly walked the two miles to my hospital from the apartment he shared with wife Dunnie. He was in his eightieth year when I first met him. He made regular visits to the hospital when we talked over the old times and he related his experiences. One of the places he had practiced was Mooseman in Saskatchewan. During the depression of the thirties, farming, particularly agricultural, was at a very low ebb throughout the continent. His many farm calls produced little income. Often a full day's work would see him returning home with some eggs, a few cabbages, maybe some spuds and half a dozen promises. There was no income from pets.

Horses were the principal workforce on the farms and became his most frequent patients. With his help as anaesthetist I operated on several 'rig' horses. In these cases one or more testicles fail to come down into the scrotum and might be found in the inguinal canal in which case you could find them by incision through the scrotum and reaching in. Others were retained inside the abdomen. Then the surgery was far more complicated, entailing a large incision in the flank, cutting through an inch or more of muscle and searching in the abdominal cavity for the problem testicle. Once found, it could usually be stretched on its attachments to the exterior and removed. The operation could take up to an hour so it was helpful not to have to supervise the anaesthetic. 'Rig' horses usually develop bad manners when they reach sexual maturity around one year old. They are cranky, mean and in fact sometimes dangerous. Many have ended up in the meat factory. The surgery fee was around $100, which in these days just about pays for a cat spay.

Doc also enabled us to get away for a visit to the UK where we stayed with relatives and old friends. He was not well versed in small animal medicine but his presence at the hospital daily could sort out the cases, determining those that should be sent up to my neighbour in Kelowna, about thirty miles away. Routine vaccinations and neuterings could await my return.

Doc lived to the ripe old age of ninety-four years. We exchanged letters every Christmas after we had left Penticton.

CHAPTER 65

Dr Huerta

Have I spelled the name properly? Do you, kind reader, recognize it as that of a medical pioneer? In the year 1936 or thereabouts the Spanish Civil War involved many more than nationals. It was a testing ground for weapons that would be used three or four years later. Many avid socialists and/or royalists joined sides to fight for a political cause, others for something exciting to do in a world that was stagnant.

Combat was fierce but sporadic. The front line was often far from medical services or hospitals. Soldiers who had sustained wounds, particularly where fractures were involved, often could not be treated for many days or even weeks. Immobilization of the damaged limb was essential. Dr Huerta conceived the idea of stripping all clothing from the part, cleaning up the wounds, aligning any broken bones as best they could and applying a plaster cast to immobilize the area.

When these casualties so treated finally arrived at base hospital, often weeks later, the cast was removed. The stench was awful, but it was found that a great deal of healing had taken place. Skin was united over wounds, good callus had joined bone ends and the patient was neither in pain nor ill.

This was a treatment used by me on many cases where dogs had sustained extensive injuries including bone fractures on the highways or through too close contact with a mowing machine. Legs that were literally hanging off were closed in plaster. The alternative treatment was amputation – not so bad in a hind limb but hard on a dog which loses a front leg.

Of the fifteen or more cases in which Dr Huerta's method was employed there was only one failure, a Pekinese whose front leg had been crushed. There was bleeding from the paw showing we had patent blood supply. After cleaning it up, clipping the hair and applying a plaster cast up to the shoulder the owner was apprised of the treatment. Written instructions were given for replacement of the cast in three weeks time. The owner returned to his home at the coast a few days later and consulted his regular veterinarian. The latter did blood tests and took X-rays, removed the cast then amputated the leg. He didn't bother to phone me.

I learned of the Peke's fate in a letter from the owner's wife telling me of this unfortunate happening. The little pet had been put to sleep because it was unable to walk owing to its physical impairment.

CHAPTER 66

Rattlers in the Okanagan

The hot, dry weather of the Okanagan which lasts from early spring until late September plus the sandy soil in many areas is very conducive to the propagation of snakes, rattlesnakes in particular. The reaction to the snake's bite depends on the amount of venom injected and hence the size of the snake. There is a rapid swelling of the bitten area. Bites around the mouth are the ones causing most distress. We had many dogs brought in after being bitten. The owners were advised that hospitalization was recommended to prevent shock – even that of the owner. We had antivenom available at $17.50 a shot but only gave it where we considered there was danger to life or the owner requested it.

Bill McCulloch brought his boxer dog in on a Sunday evening after an emergency call to my home. I met him at the hospital. The dog was bleeding from the two fang marks between the eyes. The area was puffy. I gave an injection of antivenom plus some morphine both as a sedative and to ease the local pain. The dog was kept under observation by my nurse, who had been called in for special duty.

Later that evening Bill telephoned to get a progress report, which was favourable. Then he told me that when he reached home from the hospital he found a large crowd of neighbours gathered in his garden looking at the four-foot rattlesnake which had been killed shortly after the attack. Another neighbour, Stan Gile, arrived and asked if they had killed the other one. When asked what he meant he replied, 'Well, you know they always travel in pairs.' Bill said he had never seen a crowd disappear so fast.

The effects of the bite are usually transient with the swelling subsiding within twelve hours. In California, I believe, there are different types of rattlers which can be far more toxic to both animals and humans, even causing death.

CHAPTER 67

Sailing on the Lake

Living in the small city of Penticton with a population of some 10,000 people was like being on an island in many respects. There were no near neighbours. People were more approachable, many newcomers seeking to make new friends. There was little crime. We joined the Anglican Church where June attended regularly and I sporadically. The congregation was usually sparse. At a parishioners' meeting the Reverend Eccles was asked why so few attended his services and yet the obituary column in the local paper showed burial services at St Savior's outnumbered other denominations five to one. The reverend thought a minute and then gave his answer, 'I guess we don't meet most of them until they're dead.'

I attended a council meeting and was introduced to the gathering by Mayor Matson – good advertising. I joined the riding club to get to know the horsey set. Several friends were interested in sailing. Only three or four nondescript sailboats were moored at the dock on Okanagan Lake, which had a very poor breakwater necessitating really secure mooring lines. In my second year I bought a Lightning Class nineteen-foot sailboat. June was quite happy to be my crew. With Charles Tyndal and David Boyd we formed the South Okanagan Sailing Association and organized races on Sunday afternoons when five or six boats from other parts of the lake joined us. We had no proper handicapping system so each selected his own. It wasn't satisfactory. The winds on the lake were very variable. In dead calm we puffed cigarettes then blew smoke in the air to see where our wind might come from. Then in the late afternoon a twenty-knot blow would come down one of the valleys. We would see rough water with whitecaps approaching from the distance. You had to be properly trimmed, ready and alert, as it reached you. Thirty miles to the north, still on the eighty-mile long lake, the city of Kelowna held an annual regatta which included aquatic events and sailboat races. They would have fifteen to twenty mixed types competing with similar handicapping problems. During the off

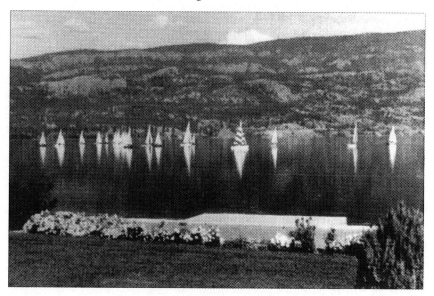

Sailing on Okanagan Lake.

season, winter, when most boats were brought up on dry land and covered over with tarps to keep off the snow, we had many discussions about our future and decided that we should all race the same class of boat. Charles was the main instigator and champion of Uffa Fox's 'Jollyboat'. This was an eighteen-foot, lightweight, drop keel, sailing dinghy designed and built in England. Its slightly faster competitor was the 'Flying Dutchman', often beaten by tactics.

We had commitments from eighteen members to buy one. They were shipped out on a freighter through the Panama Canal, trucked up from Vancouver in the early spring and prepared for racing. I called my one *Playboy*. Now I had to find an active, strong, brave young man for my crew as the racing in strong winds entailed 'hiking out'. I was lucky to find Dennis Lacey. Together we won many races and for several years enjoyed excellent sport. Other boats came from the coast to compete against us. We organized our own regatta for which local merchants were asked to donate trophies. I approached Archie Cumming for a cup. He agreed for anything up to $50. When I asked him if he thought Chart Nichol would give one he said, 'I'm sure he will. You know, for every nickel I've got, Chart has a dollar.'

We met several competitors from the State of Washington at the

Kelowna Regatta. Jim Goodfellow raced a Flying Dutchman and bemoaned the fact there was so little competition down in Wenatchee and nearby Lake Chelan. The latter was the site of the Apple Cup Derby where large racing powerboats hurled themselves around the lake at ninety miles an hour. They were sponsored by the national gasoline manufacturing companies, who were feeling the pinch at the high cost and were contemplating a pull-out. It came sooner than anyone expected. Goodfellow asked us if we would be prepared to trailer our boats down to Lake Chelan for a regatta which would have its headquarters at Campbell's lakeside Lodge. We readily agreed. On a Friday afternoon twenty-three trailered sailboats crossed the border into the US. At Campbell's arrangements had been made for those who wished to camp out in the Lodge grounds while some of us rented rooms in the Lodge.

The race committee called a meeting for 8:30 a.m. the following morning in the basement of the Medical Building. It was packed and by count we had nearly forty boats competing. Here again, working out handicaps was going to be a problem. The race committee was introduced and the chairman called on the starter to speak first.

'Well, ah understand you want a five minute gun, then a one minute gun and then a start gun. We have this little cannon that the police chief is going to set off at those times.' Apparently this had been necessary to be heard above the noisy powerboat engines. Then he went on, 'We have set up cameras at the start to ensure that no boat crosses the line before the official start. These will be on a fifteen-second exposure after the one minute gun.' By this time we were looking at one another – and winking. Next the chairman called on the 'rescue' committee for their report.

A uniformed police sergeant stood up and spoke. 'I'm goin' to have a police boat at each marker buoy. In event of a major capsize we can have a rescue helicopter over the site within five minutes.' They were prepared for the worst.

At fifteen minutes before 10:00 a.m. all competing boats were floating around the starting area – with not a breath of wind. After the final gun the first boat drifted across the starting line slowly ten minutes later. The air was thick with cigarette smoke. Half an hour later the race was called off and the boats rounded up by motor boat and towed in line back to the Lodge shore. Fortunately, the worst was over and by lunchtime a breeze had come up, which progressed into a gale by mid-afternoon when we had some great racing. We enjoyed wonderful hospitality from our hosts and we made many new friends. A hamburger barbecue, donated by the local council for all competitors, was held in the Lodge grounds on Saturday evening followed by a dance on their large patio to recorded music. Sunday was an improvement but again the morning's races were cancelled.

We came home with the satisfaction that we were now in international competition. We also started something, for some twenty years later a young Vancouver friend told me he was going to race a Laser sailboat for Canada at the Pacific International Yacht Racing Association's Regatta which was being held on the coming weekend at Lake Chelan. They expected two hundred entries.

CHAPTER 68

Bonnie Bennett

All veterinary surgeons in private practice have many amusing tales to tell. One of mine is that of the 'Incredible Journey'. The young lady we employed to open the hospital at 8:30 a.m. and admit any animals for surgery or other treatment during the morning telephoned shortly after 9:00 a.m. A very good client, Mrs Bennett, had called to say her cat had returned home that morning after being lost in Manning Park, over a hundred miles away, three weeks earlier. She and husband Fred had gone to see Jim Hume, editor of the *Penticton Herald*, to have some photographs taken and relate the whole incredible story. Hume had suggested a health check-up and an appointment was then made for me to see the cat at 10:00 a.m. At the hospital I pulled the case card and learned that 'Bonnie' was eighteen months old, had been spayed a year earlier and all vaccinations were up to date.

The Bennetts arrived and plonked a well-fleshed all black, healthy-looking cat on the examination table. They told me that when returning from Vancouver three weeks previously they had stopped in Manning Park where Bonnie had slipped out of the car and fled into the bush. Two hours searching failed to find her. That morning when their son, Clive, opened the back door to go to school Bonnie had rushed into the kitchen, gone over to her usual feeding place and started mewing. While Mrs Bennett told her story I was feeling around and was quite surprised to discover two well-developed testicles.

'Mrs Bennett,' I said, 'This is a remarkable happening but the most remarkable part of it is that she has changed her sex during the journey and is now about an eighteen-month old male cat.'

The Bennetts were flabbergasted. 'We'll be the laughing stock of the town if this gets around,' they said in dismay.

'Don't worry, I won't tell,' I reassured them. 'Just put him back in your garden and let Clive use the front door for a few days when going to school.'

Half an hour after they left Jim Hume was on the telephone to find if I had anything to add to their two-column story. 'Well Jim,' I told him, 'this isn't the first time such a remarkable journey has been reported and you can quote me. The cat is in good health, but some time when you and I are sat in a bar somewhere I will tell you the rest of the story.'

I haven't seen Jim Hume since.

CHAPTER 69

Cricket

One morning Art McKay, a well-known Naramata resident, came into my office. He was from the old country and let everybody know it by flying the Union Jack on a large flagpole in his garden. He looked very serious. He didn't have his dog with him but started off the conversation with, 'Are you a conservationist?' I sensed a request for a contribution to the 'Save the Monarchy Fund' which was getting some publicity in the National Press but it wasn't that. Next the unrelated question, 'Have you ever played cricket?' I have always been very frank about my athletic abilities, which include throwing a menacing dart and scoring goals on the soccer pitch but beyond that I am a duffer.

'No,' I said. 'I've dressed up in white pants and shirt and stood out on a hot field with ten other uniformed chaps who had nothing better to do. I can't say I enjoyed it and certainly didn't do very well. What can I do for you, Art?'

'Well,' he said, a little bit crestfallen, 'Our side is short one player for next Sunday's match against St. George's School in Vernon [a town about forty miles north of Penticton]. If we can't field a team it will be the end of cricket in the Okanagan Valley. Possibly also in the interior of British Columbia.'

The strains of 'There'll Always be an England' drifted through my mind. Was I to be the means of ending a truly British institution, to have my name coupled with an event in history that would be told over the port wine and cheese when elder ex-pats reminisced about the gradual demise of the Empire? No, I could not let that happen. I told Art I wasn't much good, having a serious lack of co-ordination which I felt was a very necessary qualification in such a demanding game, but he wouldn't be deterred. After further remonstrations I agreed to be picked up on the following Sunday morning at 10:00 a.m. and was reminded to bring a lunch. There followed a search for white boots and white longs, both of which were in short supply. David Boyd phoned the next day to tell me that the word had gone round that a Hampshire cricketer of some distinction would be joining the team for Sunday's game. David had a spare pair of white pants which he would be very happy to lend me. A pair of white 'sneakers' would suffice for boots.

Throughout life I have not been able to sleep well if a major problem confronted me. It happened when I had undertaken to repair an umbilical hernia in a colt worth $10,000. It happened before all my professional exams. It happened when I was to appear before a magistrate charged with reckless control of an automobile, and it happened as I confronted the prospect of getting a duck at my first Canadian cricket game.

The fateful day arrived. On Sunday morning about six of us piled into one station wagon while a second one took the remainder of the team plus the bats, leg pads, cricket balls and some sort of scoring numbers. We were on our way.

The school resembled others I had known in my infancy. The boys wore gray pants, blazers with a crest on the breast pocket and little caps on their heads. The game was due to start at 1:00 p.m. so there would be time for lunch, and beer. I learned later that fortification prior to a game was the normal *modus operandi* – a handicap as it were. For this purpose a plentiful supply of beer had been brought along. It would be dispensed to the team members for a dollar a bottle and consumed in a surreptitious manner out of Delft mugs. Maybe it would help.

This was a British type of private school, quite distinct from the 'free' government ones. It was supported by hefty fees. The team we were up against comprised boys between thirteen and sixteen years old, well dressed in whites and exuding confidence.

A number of parents and local supporters sat in deck chairs close to the pavilion. We lost the toss and the school team batted first. From the performance of our fielders I soon learned there were no stars. The boys sent our bowling for fours and occasional sixes. The number of catches dropped were an embarrassment. Perhaps most of our team had been co-opted by Art using the same approach he had used on me.

The boys did well, scoring some 117 runs for only eight wickets – and then declared – no, I won't explain either the rules or the language, it's better that you don't know.

Along came the tea break and some nice sandwiches provided by the school's kitchen, giving us an opportunity to meet some of the parents and assure them the game engendered sportsmanship and great skill in their offspring. Then it was our turn to bat. I would like to tell a story in which we nearly equalled the opponents' score with only five runs needed. Then I, as last man, was called in to bat – and with a mighty swipe sent the ball flying over the pavilion to score six runs and win the match. But it wasn't so. Art and Lyle, the first batsmen, were soon dispatched. Boyd held up well until called out lbw. Jackson hit his own wicket and sent the bails flying and the rest crumbled for 37 runs when it came my turn. Could I save the day? No, I couldn't. I survived three balls but the fourth one sneaked through and took the middle stump. It was all over.

On the way home we pulled off the highway at a viewpoint and gazed out on the placid lake strangely calm in the evening setting sun, and finished the beer. The demise of cricket in the valley was assured on that Sunday afternoon. But who knows? There may be other McKays who will come along with the same enthusiasm as my old friend.

CHAPTER 70

Von Brevern of the Mounted Police

One evening as it was nearly dusk I was stopped at the traffic light going south on Main Street at Eckhart Avenue. Just as the light turned green, allowing me to proceed, a car swept in front of me and turned right to go down Eckhart Avenue. It was a police car. I blared on my horn as I went forward. Annoyed, I travelled on but soon became aware of a siren and the flashing red light of a police car following. I pulled to the side and stopped. An RCMP constable approached the driver's side window, which I lowered.

'May I see your driving licence, sir,' he commenced. After he handed it back to me he said, 'Are you aware that you are travelling after lighting up time with only the car's sidelights on?'

I replied, 'No, constable, I wasn't, but I can soon rectify that,' as I switched the lights on.

Next he took out a notebook and said, 'I will have to charge you for an offence under the Motor Vehicle Act.'

I asked, 'What is your name, constable?'

He replied, 'Von Brevern.'

'Well,' I said, 'we will go to the police station where you can write out your charge and I can write mine. I am charging you with the reckless operation of a motor vehicle by turning in front of a moving vehicle without any sign, without using your siren and in contravention of regulations pertaining to police pursuit. Now make your choice – but I assure you the penalty for me will be minimal while the blemish on your record will be permanent and damning.'

He thought for a moment, closed his notebook, said, 'Drive carefully, sir,' then he returned to his car and drove off.

On a sunny day in early summer I was returning from a visit in Oliver some sixteen miles south of Penticton. There was little traffic as I sailed along in my station wagon, probably doing 50 mph. I took my foot off the accelerator as I entered the outskirts of Okanagan Falls to slow down going through the village. But it wasn't enough. At the far end an RCMP constable stood in the road beckoning me to

189

pull to the side. It was my old 'friend', von Brevern. He asked to see my driving licence then produced his book. After writing for a minute or so he handed me a ticket with the words, 'You are charged with operating a motor vehicle in a 30 mph zone whilst travelling at 43 mph. Your speed was recorded by radar at the entrance to the village.' I told him I did not see any sign indicating a speed limit but had slowed down at the first buildings and was surely doing no more than 20 mph when he stopped me. Then I drove off.

But it bothered me as I was a careful driver and always (well, mostly) obeyed highway signs. That evening I drove down to Okanagan Falls and retraced my approach to the village. There was no speed limit sign. I parked the car then walked the side of the highway and found the sign lying in the ditch. Next morning I phoned the police station, reached von Brevern, and requested him to meet me at the Falls at noon – where I showed him the sign and said I would contest the charge on the grounds that the 'radar trap' had not been properly set up. He said he could not withdraw the charge. The local paper printed an item that fifteen motorists who had been caught in the same trap had been fined $30 each.

Three weeks later I appeared at the Oliver courthouse to answer the charge, which was presented by a police sergeant in the red Mountie tunic accompanied by von Brevern and another constable. The presiding magistrate was a very aged local orchardist who seemingly suffered from both a sight and a hearing impairment – and also a mental one, as I was about to discover. After all the evidence was presented I told my side of the story and asked that the charge be dismissed. The 'beak' said that although the sign was gone I should have known there was a speed limit. He found me guilty as charged and fined me $75 because I was a veterinary doctor and he felt the punishment should be in accordance with one's ability to pay.

I told him I could not accept his decision and would appeal to a more experienced judge for a fair hearing. This annoyed him and he told me that I would have to make a deposit of $200 if I intended to appeal, also that the deposit would have to be made or the fine paid at his court within one week.

Of course he was wrong in all three areas, as I learned later, but we were booked to fly to Britain on the following day so when I reached home I wrote out and mailed a cheque to the old buzzard for the $75.

On my return from holiday I wrote a scathing letter to the *Vancouver Sun* newspaper about local magistrates and the miscarriage of justicc, with a copy to the Attorney General of British Columbia. They were all removed from the bench within four months then replaced with lawyers appointed by the Department of Justice.

CHAPTER 71

Hugh Gough

One of my favourite clients was Hugh Gough, an old Englishman in his seventy-fourth year, who kept two aging cocker spaniels. He lived in a small house on what I think was called Power Street, quite near to the Hockey Arena, which was also the venue for the annual craft fair. This was handy for Hugh as one of his hobbies was cooking – baking bread, making jam and other preserves plus a very palatable red wine, all of which became the currency of our transactions and also won him many prizes.

Hugh rode a large tricycle around town to do his shopping but had no way of bringing his pets to my hospital. House calls were the order of the day when he needed my services. Whenever we had a slack day I would phone Hugh and say I was sending my groomer to pick up his dogs and have them groomed, bathed, and de-flead. We did this three or four times a year and I always brought the dogs back to him. At this time we would have lots to talk about. His gratitude was expressed by a gift of an assortment of jam, pickles, preserves, and of course, a couple of bottles of his wine. June was very sceptical of his culinary hygiene and left the consumption to me.

Hugh was a member of the Canadian Legion. He had a collection of German memorabilia which he had brought back after the 1914 war, including bayonets and a Luger pistol. He had taken the lot in a large cardboard box to a Legion meeting intending to donate all of it. When told that they didn't want that junk he carried the box out with tears in his eyes. He never went back.

Then the time came when I was leaving Penticton. I called to say goodbye. Hugh said how much he had appreciated my services and asked if there was anything at all in his house that I would like. I said, 'Yes, the Luger pistol.'

'Well, you shall have it. I will put that in my will,' he promised.

Fully two years later a friend told me that Hugh had died several months previously. There was no Luger pistol. A few weeks later I wrote a letter to the Attorney General's Department requesting a copy of Hugh's will. Sure enough, one paragraph stated: 'I wish my Luger pistol to be given to my good friend, Dr Earnshaw, for his kindness to me and my dogs.'

The will had been probated by a Penticton resident and approved by a local lawyer who knew me well and could easily have contacted me. I wrote a letter to him expressing my concern, adding that if I failed to receive a reply within ten days the matter would be taken up 'in another place'. This brought a reply by return full of apology adding that matters would be put right immediately. I was asked to attend the local cop shop where I obtained a permit to own the Luger and it was subsequently brought down to my residence by an RCMP constable. Good old Hugh.

CHAPTER 72

Lake Pennask

The Callaghans were near neighbours. We visited back and forth regularly. They had a growing family like ours. Howard Callaghan was a member of a local law firm and keen on outdoor activities including fishing, a sport in which I hoped to improve my knowledge.

One of my clients whom I shall call Brock owned a fishing camp at Pennask Lake, which was fifteen miles or more back in the hills above Peachland. It had a reputation for producing trout to one or two pounds but no whoppers. The camp consisted of six or seven Army bell type tents renting for $10 a night. In front of each was a fireplace with wood and a picnic table with benches. Row boats and canoes, pulled up on the beach, were available to rent for a further $10 per day. Brock stayed up there throughout the spring and summer for as long as his customers continued to come. It was a lonely life but made more bearable by the company of two cocker spaniels – which is where I come into the picture.

My services varied from removing porcupine quills, deeply imbedded fishhooks, speargrass lodged in the ears of the dogs, to Brock's instructions to shear them, all over – and close. This, before he went up in the spring.

The greatest difficulty was getting there via an old poorly maintained logging road winding through the heavily wooded hills and swamps. Where the latter were bad, lengths of alder three or four inches thick were laid close together over the worst areas, a so-called corduroy road bed.

A part of my reward for services rendered was an invitation to take a friend up any time and use the facilities without charge. This is where Howie Callaghan comes in.

We planned to go up there after work, which would be when his law office could dispense with his services. We took my station wagon loaded with fishing gear, sleeping bags, food, a Coleman propane stove and a bottle of rum – to share with Brock. Leaving

Penticton around 6:00 p.m., it was nearly 8:00 p.m. when we reached the camp after a rough trip. Brock greeted us warmly. We would get in at least an hour's fishing for it was well into September. We took a rowing boat and had two rods out while one of us rowed. We had spinners, flies and worms plus a landing net. It was amazing. A fish was no sooner hauled in than there was a strike on the other rod. All the fish were better than one pound, some nearly two. Well before dark we had fourteen nice trout so we went in to organize our sleeping arrangements.

Brock had supplied straw pallets for which we were glad. The coffeepot was put on while we sat at the table, brought out the rum, and listened to the fascinating stories of a real bushman.

Across the lake nestled in the trees was a large building which we learned was the rural clubhouse for a most exclusive membership. It was also the building where Prince Philip and Queen Elizabeth would stay a few years later.

Breakfast at 5:30 a.m. was shared with whiskey jacks, little grey birds which hopped all over the table sharing our bacon, eggs and toast. The lake was very still with a light mist rising from the placid waters. We packed up our food supplies into the large cardboard box then wrapped Howie's sleeping bag around it to ensure any marauding chipmunks would not smell the food and come hunting it. Then we launched the dinghy for some more fishing. It was equally good. Before 8:00 a.m. we left, after evicting three or four chipmunks which had chewed their way through Howie's brand new sleeping bag then into the cardboard box and were enjoying the remnants of the apple pie. By 9:00 a.m. we were back in Penticton, each with a dozen beautiful rainbow trout.

I made a promise that one day I would return to Pennask Lake. There's time yet.

CHAPTER 73

Tragic Loss

On a Saturday morning about 11:00 o'clock there was a loud explosion or crash which was heard all over the city. The clients in my office speculated as to the cause but came nowhere near the tragic news broadcast from the CJOR Radio Station at noon. 'It is with great regret and sadness we announce that an airplane crash occurred at the Penticton Airport this morning when two planes collided then fell to the ground. All members of the Parmley family plus the pilots of both planes have been killed. A further report will follow at 1:00 p.m.'

Dick Parmley was one of the leading citizens and personalities of the city. He owned the Esso fuel distribution facility for the whole area, which included that for motors and home heating. He also had cattle on leased land above the West Bench. Apparently, Imperial Oil had sent two of their executives to Penticton in the ten-seater aircraft. The Parmley family were offered a joy ride over the area whilst the businessmen did their company work. Dick was happy to take his wife and children.

The tragedy caused a pall of sadness. Many social and sporting events were cancelled for the next week.

CHAPTER 74

Wine Making

The garden at our new residence boasted several fruit trees of different variety and an area for vegetable growing, plus two mature grape vines – red and green. Local folklore had it that by far the best fertilizer and source of nitrogen was a dead pussycat buried close by the roots. Visualizing a bountiful crop in the fall I complied with the suggestion when the victim of a street accident came to the hospital for disposal.

Next, with the harvest almost ready, it was necessary to go to the horse's mouth and learn the intricacies of the wine making process. My tutor was Captain Temple of Summerland who had been a resident of the area for many years and surely knew all the ins and outs of the vintner. It was easier than I thought.

'You just get a five-gallon earthenware crock, put your grapes in to half fill it and crush them with a wooden pole. Then add water up to three quarters full, cover the whole thing with some curtain material to keep the flies out, and don't go near it for six weeks,' was his readily given advice. We had enough grapes to set up two crocks, one for red wine and the other for white. They were placed in a corner of the basement.

Three weeks later June called my attention to a constant humming noise in the kitchen. I checked the light switches for a short and the portable radio for something – then I opened the door to the basement. The hum was much louder. When we went down the stairs we were aware of a virtual cloud of fruit flies which had been attracted to the grape odour and found their way in somehow. The crocks were moved to the garage for the remainder of the process.

Captain Temple had to be consulted for the next step. Again he made it clear that the process was simple by telling me over the telephone, 'Well, you just get your bottles ready and use a funnel after you have removed all the crud and scum from above the wine. You can use the curtain material as a filter. Hammer your corks in well and give the wine another couple of weeks before you sample it.'

Two weeks later all we had was vinegar. The bottles had been brought into the basement by this time, the colder weather having eliminated the fruit flies. This time we went to a different 'expert'. This one had apparently produced a palatable vintage but had no samples to prove it. He told us, 'You will have to decant some of the wine and add sugar to remove the tartness.' This involved pulling all the corks but we managed it one evening. We had about eight bottles of each colour which should satisfy every palate at Thanksgiving and maybe also at Christmas.

Some time later June told me she had heard several popping noises coming from the basement but hadn't thought anything about it. When we went down to ascertain the source the basement floor was a mess – wet with both red and white wine as nearly all the bottles had popped their corks and spilled most of the contents. The process was a disaster never to be repeated.

Some time later I spoke to Captain Temple at a riding club meeting. When I recounted our sad experience he said nonchalantly, 'Well, you know, I never actually made the stuff meself.'

CHAPTER 75

Fruit

The Okanagan Valley is ideally suited to fruit growing. The economic value of this industry has been like a roller coaster. The lifestyle of the orchardist is generally good but very dependant on a willingness to work hard and long hours when necessary and suffer the vagaries of weather and prices, which together may mean the difference between solvency, prosperity and, unfortunately, bankruptcy.

I have not been intimately connected with the fruit industry but will relate a few stories that have come my way.

Economic conditions in the thirties were no less severe in the valley than elsewhere. Orchardists had the means to grow much of the family's food, but paying the taxes, driving the tractors and car, plus clothing the kids necessitated cash income. Prices were down on everything and Penticton was at that time very isolated from population centres where fruit might have a better chance of being sold.

Many orchardists would pack up boxes of apples then send them by rail at low cost to remote towns with larger populations in British Columbia and Alberta with a note attached to the station manager: 'Please sell these apples then send the receipts to me at Box 274, Penticton, BC. Thanks. John Jones.'

The Cawston and Keremeos area farmers were overjoyed when a big American canning company announced that they would be buying field tomatoes at the end of the growing season. In the spring, pasture was ploughed up and seed put in. There is no better place to grow such tasty tomatoes, some of which reach grapefruit size. The current price was ten cents a pound at harvest time, which portended to be a bonanza. Frowns became smiles as the farmers saw a bumper crop developing. The frowns returned when the company buyers came back at harvest time and announced that the price would be three cents a pound, barely enough to cover the production costs. Committees were set up to represent the growers.

While deliberations continued for many days the crop sat on the ground with the possibility of becoming over-ripe and worthless.

Finally the day was saved when the buying price was settled at six cents a pound then the crop harvested.

A committee studied the problem more carefully and submitted a resolution to the company. A separate contract would be signed with each grower on the basis, 'Ten cents a pound or no seed in the ground.' It worked for several years.

Marketing conditions were such that buyers would arrive at harvest time to buy apples, the main crop that would appear in the supermarkets for months to come. Prices offered by the wholesalers varied according to variety, appearance and texture. It was a haphazard process and left many growers feeling they had not been dealt with fairly.

In the 1950s, probably the best time of all, a company was formed called B.C. Tree Fruits Ltd. It took all fruit, housed it in spacious warehouses, then marketed it in an orderly manner, securing fair and standard prices.

It was mandatory to belong, then adhere to a set of rules which precluded private sales, taking truckloads of fruit to the coast or having individual fruit stands where the orchardist had the potential for direct sales to the public. All of these conditions were moderated in time. As fruit was graded for quality before sale it became necessary to employ a large labour force most of whom were wives, daughters or cousins of the growers. The duration of employment was usually fourteen weeks which then allowed for unemployment benefits over the next few months.

The quality of fruit sold improved and the headache of selling was removed. Large surpluses of misshapen or bruised fruit were salvaged for juice. A local paper published a photograph of a 'mountain' of pears which had been rejected for sale. I wrote to the Capozzi winery in Kelowna and described a product I had known in the UK. Made from pears it was a champagne called 'Babycham'. It was marketed in eight-ounce bottles and became a favourite ladies' drink. They were not able to undertake the process but sent me a crate of twelve bottles of their best wines in appreciation of the suggestion.

One of the popular restaurants on Main Street served the most delicious apple pie which became the favourite dessert for many locals. Neither the staff nor the manager would divulge the variety of fruit used which would have been a great asset to local cooks. It became a subject of discussion as such a secret might even be an advantage in the pie baking competition at the annual Fall Fair. One of my clients had been a cook at the restaurant. I persuaded him to tell me the secret on condition that I would not divulge it. As that was forty years ago I feel free to tell you what he said. 'The apple pulp all comes from China in five-gallon drums.'

In mid October, Premier Bennett favoured the city with a visit during which he held a cabinet meeting in the City Hall. It was the evening that a deputation representing fruit growers was to be received to relate their grievances. There was quite a crowd of them. The spokesman addressed the Premier, 'Mr Premier, you will no doubt be surprised at the number of fruit growers who have come here tonight to tell you of the sad state of our industry.'

'Yes, I am,' said the Premier, 'I thought you'd all be in California by now.'

CHAPTER 76

Ted Pendergraft

One of the more prosperous ranchers was Ted Pendergraft of Osoyoos, which is at the south end of the Okanagan Valley bordering on the United States. It boasts numerous orchards and an area of true desert, an extension of the Arizona desert which crops up in several states and contains similar fauna and flora.

Ted lived in the village with his wife and several sons. This was home base with some horse stabling but he ran cattle both to the east and the west of town. I had met Ted when called upon to do inspections on behalf of the Federal or Provincial Government. He was very knowledgeable of veterinary matters so I was surprised when he called me to attend a heifer which was unable to calve. This was because I knew Ted was a capable man who had probably done difficult calf deliveries as often as I had. But now he wanted me to do a caesarian section to possibly save the calf and probably the mother which was really too young and small to have been bred. I took all I needed and went down on a Monday morning. The heifer had been brought in from the range to home base. I recall that a sedative was given, then a paralumbar nerve block. The operation was undertaken with the help of Ted and his several sons. When I asked Ted to fetch me more hot water he referred the task to son Ronnie. Ted had watched diligently, asking questions about each step of the operation, which I was quite happy to answer. Both mother and offspring survived. I only did one more similar operation for him. I heard from nearby ranchers that Ted had done several successfully himself. A few years later he told me he only operated on his own stock.

CHAPTER 77

We Move to the Coast

I did not enjoy the Okanagan winters. The outside work was hard on a person. I longed to be near the sea. Our life had become repetitious and we weren't making a lot of money. I decided it was time for another move. Several drug salesmen had told me that Dr Ian Bruce was terribly busy in North Vancouver and badly needed some extra help. I had met Ian at one of the Association meetings and liked him. I wrote and suggested that, as I was contemplating a move, it might be to our mutual advantage to join forces. His reply was tardy but came as a telephone call to my office, 'Be pleased to see you anytime.'

Another veterinarian was anxious to buy my hospital so a deal was struck and once again I was 'on the loose'. I came down to the coast and made an appointment to meet Ian at his office. He didn't show up. I looked around the area, which seemed like a nice place to live, so made a second appointment. Again he didn't show up. Several empty stores were available for rent in the area so I decided to have my own place. I rented an empty store and employed a carpenter to erect partitions to provide a spacious waiting room, examination room, office, operating room, kennel room and storage area. The work was to be completed within three weeks when my $400 deposit would be supplemented to meet all bills. Then I returned to Penticton and took June and the two boys for a holiday on the Oregon Coast. When I returned to inspect the work on the new office nothing had been done. I never saw my carpenter again. I had selected him through a telephone number in the employment section of the local paper. The number was 'no longer in service'.

I was hoping to open on 1 June, just ten days away. This time I went to a house and interviewed a second carpenter, Bob McCombie, who came to the store, looked at the job and told me he couldn't start for three days but would finish it in three, allowing me to come in and paint what he had already built. My drugs and instruments were scheduled to be delivered as soon as the place was ready. June was the receptionist and between us we each put in twelve-hour days, furnishing, cleaning, buying supplies and just getting ready.

On 1 June 1963 we opened the 'Lonsdale Veterinary Clinic'.

CHAPTER 78

Back in the Big City

We were going through the same thing all over again – and it was exciting. This time it was ninety-five per cent small animal practice and for a while horse work, mainly floating teeth on a Sunday morning. The help was often a teen-aged girl whose parents were wise enough to give her something animate to love – and keep her attention away from the boys – a procedure I have approved of in many places. But the cost of maintaining stabling, buying hay and suitable attire were often such a strain that the veterinarian's bills were ignored for months.

After the pets were providing a reasonable income I stopped doing horse work and gave the owners the phone number of a colleague in Surrey, twenty-five miles away, who could take care of them. One previous client, Percy Williamson, who kept Arab horses in Kelowna, asked me to fly up once a month and check on his very valuable show animals. This took most of the morning. After a pleasant lunch with Percy he would lend me a car to drive down to see old friends in Penticton then leave it at the Kelowna airport when I caught the 8:00 p.m. flight back to the coast. This was a full day's trip for which the fee was $250, including airfare, but my work at the clinic became more important so I soon had to forego that day's outing.

One lady came to me with a spaniel suffering from seborrheic dermatitis which responded well to a product called Protamone D, which came from the US. Strangely, no pharmaceutical firm in Canada supplied it so I had to travel across the border and purchase supplies from a veterinarian there. The dog's owner was Doris Orr. She was very concerned at the indiscriminate breeding of pets which subsequently could not be found homes. She and a few helpers regularly put on garage sales and other money-raising efforts then subsidized the cost of spaying both cats and dogs for those who could not afford the normal fee. I agreed to give a price reduction on all cases she referred to my office, which was the best client builder I could have had and lasted until I retired, nearly thirty years later.

Those that I spayed came back for vaccinations and subsequent health care. In later years I helped her publish the *Kitty Letter*, which gave reports of her work to far off places and enhanced her charity income.

I have always felt it most important for a professional person in business to get 'known'. I attended Council meetings, joined the Kiwanis Club, and became a member of the North Vancouver Players, a repertory group with whom I appeared in several plays. I helped Alderman Suttis plan the local theatre, Don Poole the Community Concerts and Ann MacDonald to found the Community Arts Council, and I became chairman of the North Shore Traffic Safety Committee.

I did not become political within the Veterinary Association but did join the Veterinary Academy, a group of practitioners which met regularly to hear speakers on various academic subjects. When in Penticton I had attended a few Association meetings and was appointed in charge of public relations. I was aware that there was a deplorable lack of knowledge in the pet owning public regarding vaccination amongst other things. I solicited all the companies supplying vaccine within the Province and asked them to contribute financially to an advertising programme through the daily press in relation to the percentage of their estimated sales in BC. The target was $5000. The council was informed of my programme but, rather than support the effort, told me that our profession did not advertise. Although I pointed out that no single practitioner was involved, they asked me to return the funds already collected. Nowadays, of course, flea medicines, prescription diets and heartworm pills are on every television programme.

When the annual meeting was held in Penticton I organized the gathering, which was to be a business meeting followed by a dinner and dance on the *Sycamous*, a paddle wheel steamer which had plied the lake for many years and was now beached as a tourist attraction. I solicited all the drug and instrument companies for spot prizes to be given at the dance. The response was excellent – but I was told later by a council member that it was unprofessional conduct. Now, of course, they can't get enough from the companies, even extending to a hospitality room where one can 'tie one on' at no cost.

CHAPTER 79

Mainly Small Animal Practice

When we came to North Vancouver in 1963 we lived in a rented house for one year. We were subsidized by monthly payments from the sale of the Penticton Veterinary Hospital, also by rents from the house there. Business was excellent. When we were in a position to buy our own place we selected one not far from the clinic with downstairs accommodation which could be used for night-time examinations of pets after office hours. June had been replaced with a succession of nurses and was busy with the housework, entertaining friends and expecting our third child. We enjoyed fishing and sailing when time permitted. Two years later I bought a building about two miles away which had previously housed a medical clinic. It was well equipped with examination rooms, sinks, office space and waiting room. All I had to add was a spacious kennel room to provide inside runs that could be hosed down.

We held a monthly luncheon of all the six veterinarians practicing on the North Shore. Between us we devised a plan which would have only two of us on call at weekends and one at night during the week. It worked well and gave us free time which had been unheard of previously. Later, with the advent of emergency clinics, our telephones were switched to their number at 6:00 p.m. on weekdays and 1:00 p.m. on Saturdays.

Before long we were grossing more in a month than Penticton had garnered in a year. We needed a further veterinarian and I was lucky to get an enthusiastic young man, Keith Lilley, from England. He took over the Lonsdale Clinic while I built up the new office which I called Highlands Animal Hospital.

It was located in Edgemont Village, the centre of a salubrious residential area. I scouted around to find a property on which we could build a nice home and, through a client, found an acre of land fronting on Capilano Road, a desirable location, which was occupied by an aging couple. I went to see Hugh Brown who lived in a very old but charming one-storey wooden building at the back of the property.

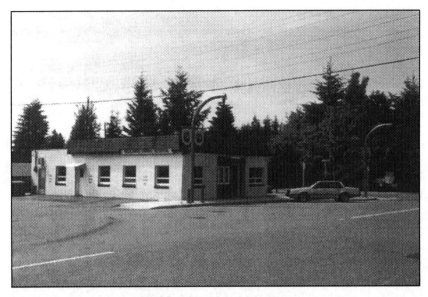

Highlands Animal Hospital.

There were huge fir trees bordering the driveway leading down to it. He told me a real estate company had wanted to buy the place a few years earlier but could not meet his price of $30,000. I didn't know if I could either so I said, 'Hugh, I will give you a deposit of $50 for an exclusive option to purchase the property on or before April 1, two months hence, the money to be forfeited if I fail to complete.'

He agreed and I put this in writing with a copy to each of us. I was delighted then wondered where I would raise the cash. An acre of land is a lot to maintain. I felt that if I got the rear half-acre with a driveway down the side and could be screened from the road noise by a couple of houses it would still suit me well.

I went to the planning department at Municipal Hall and with their help mentally subdivided the acre into two lots bordering on the road with a fifteen-foot entrance to a driveway that would reach the half acre and house at the back. This concept was presented to council and approved. Next I saw my lawyer and briefed him on my proposals. I would sell the front half for $22,000 and complete that sale in the morning of 1 April. I would then borrow $10,000 from the bank and be back in his office at 3:00 p.m. to meet Brown and conclude his deal. I asked him to ensure that the parties involved would be there on time

The best offer I got for the two lots was $20,000 but felt that would be adequate. On 1 April everything went according to plan. The papers were signed in the morning. The bank gave me a draft for ten thousand at lunchtime and I happily looked forward to increasing my estate before tea time. Then Brown failed to show up. There was no reply to the repeated phone calls I made, but at 8:00 p.m. he called me. 'There's two men out on the front of the property measuring the land. They tell me they own it.'

'Well, Hugh,' I pacified him. 'We expected you in the lawyer's office at 3:00 p.m. but you didn't make it. I will send a taxi over to your house in the morning at 10:00 a.m. and then meet you in Mr MacDonald's office fifteen minutes later. Don't worry about it and tomorrow you'll have the $30,000.'

Brown was given a month to vacate. He was happy to have the money with which he intended to take his wife to Scotland for a holiday. They were both in their early eighties. Meanwhile the two builders were forging ahead with two houses. It cost me $1,000 to relocate the water, sewer mains and electricity down the driveway but I was delighted. I found a good tenant for the property and was quite happy to leave its development until later.

During this period when necessary we hired extra help which afforded us time for return visits to England and I also went to Australia to visit my brother Desmond, who had emigrated several years earlier with his family and now worked in government service.

When everything seemed rosy, Keith announced that he was anxious to have his own practice and would be happy to purchase the Lonsdale office.

CHAPTER 80

Move to the Country – and Back

Keith was an excellent assistant. A year earlier I had taken him in as full partner, allowing him to owe me the purchase price over a period of time. I knew he would be a good neighbour while his business acumen would ensure the repayment of the loans. I therefore agreed to sell him his office, which further added to his indebtedness.

By now I had four offspring. Richard, aged eighteen, had left school and moved out of the house to conform to one of my rules. He was making enough money in a landscaping job to pay rent and feed himself. John, at sixteen, was attending a private school some thirty miles away. Keri was twelve and eagerly looked forward to horseback riding. Sheri, just turning five, was about to enter kindergarten. We decided to move to the country. We divided our house into an upstairs apartment for renting while the basement would give us a separate spacious apartment should we wish to stay in town overnight.

We found a suitable property at Langley, about thirty miles inland, with a spacious Tudor style house on three acres, having a double garage, barn, duck pond and small orchard located in a quiet area. I employed a young assistant, Neil Cropper, to manage the hospital while I would come into town on a Tuesday to do mainly surgery. In the evening I would play bridge with friends and stay overnight in the apartment.

June was not happy with the move, missing many friends and her church, which had become a big factor in her life.

Before long we had a mare with foal. Keri was riding well in the spacious riding ring I had built, Sheri had started school, and the addition of four sheep, six chickens and two rabbits added to the country scene. John was at high school doing well on the rugby team and working part time at a drive-in restaurant. But it wasn't to last. The separation of our ways was becoming a worrying problem. Then Dr Cropper told me he wanted to move elsewhere. And so after one

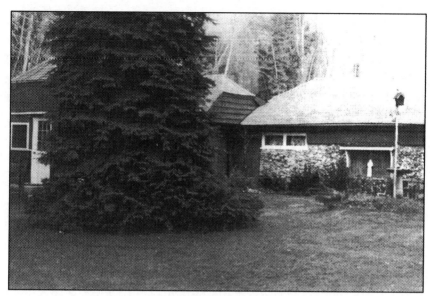

The old cottage.

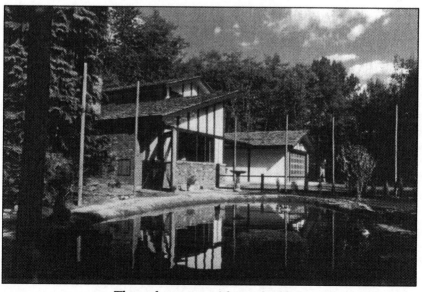

The replacement with pond added.

year, which I should call a sabbatical, we moved back to our North Vancouver house and I was again working full time.

It was a disappointment for me and for the children. We settled into the routines we had left behind a year earlier. Our domestic situation was deteriorating as our pursuits became separate. My free time was spent with male friends, fishing and playing golf or taking the children out. Before long my wife and I were occupying separate bedrooms.

The old house I had bought earlier became vacant and I decided to move there with some of the household furniture. There was a lot of work to be done both inside and outside the house. This kept me occupied. I had not seen the family for a few weeks when surprisingly the vicar of St. Catherine's Church called to meet 'the new resident'. We had a long chat which showed me I was mistaken in shutting myself off from the children who would presume I was upset with them. I readily made amends and took them out to dinner. After this June regularly brought them over in her car, dropping them off at the driveway entrance. An additional bedroom and spacious outside deck were built and the grounds tidied up. My friends came to Saturday evening parties. Bridge games, my involvement with the Kiwanis Club and municipal affairs in addition to a busy practice kept me fully occupied. A year later Keri, my elder daughter, joined me. Then along came Sport.

CHAPTER 81

Sport

Small animal or pet practice was becoming very much routine and more rewarding financially each year. The newer drugs and equipment made diagnosis and treatment easier and more successful. The new emergency clinics springing up in most cities took care of calls between 6:00 p.m. and 8:00 a.m. the next morning and throughout weekends from 1:00 p.m. on Saturdays. Referral hospitals were opening, where a veterinarian with a specialist degree in one particular field, be it surgery, dermatology, urology or gastro-intestinal problems, could come to one's aid with a second opinion should a case be puzzling or beyond one's ability to effect a cure.

Then there were the oddball cases. Mrs Godwin arrived one morning with a large elderly black labrador already showing a few white ones around his muzzle. She held him in check with a stout leather leash as he pulled her around the waiting room to explore a cat basket held on the lap of another client. His tail wagged rapidly suggesting a pussycat therein. He made a little bark. Tina, my receptionist, wisely suggested to Mrs Godwin that he should be brought into the examination room at once with apologies to the cat owner who readily agreed. I was summoned by buzzer from the back – three short buzzes which said, 'Hurry up.'

I was introduced to Sport who seemed ill at ease, tugging first one way then the other. Mrs Godwin was sitting down and holding on grimly.

'Doctor,' she stated, 'I am ashamed to be here. I have not had a good night's sleep for six months since my husband passed away. Sport and he were very attached to each other. Now he just howls all night. I have kept the radio on and used heavy drapes over the windows to dull the noise. Fortunately the neighbours have never complained but it's making me ill and I want you to put him to sleep.'

Putting a healthy pet to sleep is anathema to me – unless it's a biter. By this time I had just moved into the old house on Capilano

Road and felt I could take care of him. For me, labs are the most companionable of all canines.

'Mrs Godwin,' I said, 'I couldn't do so to such a fine animal, but I will adopt him myself and give him a good home. I will send you a note in a month's time to let you know how we are getting on – and there will be no charge.'

Mrs Godwin was crying freely then left mumbling her thanks. Sport was taken through to the kennel room and put into a spacious cage, the door of which had stout aluminum bars. I carried on with my routine work. I was preparing to go for lunch when one of the nurses came to my office.

'Sport has chewed the bars of his cage and is loose in the kennel room,' she told me. 'What should we do with him?'

I went back with her. Sure enough he was loose. The cage door lay on the cement floor twisted like a pretzel. Sport was looking up at me, wagging his tail and looking proud of himself, obviously not aware that he had done some $185 worth of damage. I secured a chain leash and attached it to his collar and then put him in one of the indoor exercise runs, each of which had a sloping concrete floor down to a drain at the far end. The near end of the chain, which was two yards long, was clipped into the chain link of the six-foot high door. When I came back after lunch I found he had in some way lifted the heavy chain link door in its metal frame off its hinges and had dragged it the nearly twenty yard length of the kennel room. I left him there until it was going-home time where, with his stout leather leash firmly gripped, we went for a long walk through the forested area of Capilano Park. When any other dog was seen his hackles rose and it was all I could do to restrain him from an attack.

Back at the house I prepared a good meal for both of us then we sat in the sparsely furnished sitting room waiting for an employee from the telephone company to arrive and do some wiring to keep us in touch. About 8:00 p.m. a young bearded man appeared at the French doors. Sport made a wild lunge, crashing into and smashing several glass panes. The young man disappeared rapidly. This was when I broke the first walking stick across his back. He slept in the house and after a walk in the morning I left him inside. When I came home at lunchtime he greeted me warmly. I found all the curtains had been pulled down from their attachments. I started on the second walking stick. We carried on for days like that. Long walks, good food, lots of love and frequent chastisement. Then I took him to the hospital and neutered him. The change was rapid. After only a few weeks he became placid, took little notice of other dogs and could be left in the house without wrecking things.

By this time I had completely fenced the garden, which was very private, and made him a comfortable resting place in the garage for daytime. He had a nice bed in the house for nights. We enjoyed our long morning walks in a wooded area nearby and on several afternoons in winter I took him duck shooting down at the shore in Ladner.

A good friend offered to come and feed him if I was away for days at a time, to which he was quite amenable. When we needed to have some work done on the house I used a long chain clipped onto his collar then tied at the other end securely beside his day place in the double garage. The workmen could come and go without interference. The chain gave him a radius of some eighteen feet. When I came home for lunch I found he had chewed everything within reach in the garage, including a vigorous attack on my lawnmower.

But it was all worth it. I loved that dog. In writing these words I have a lump in my throat and a tear in my eye. Time passed. He was slowing down. It became a sorrowful parting when we left him in charge of a friend while I took a three-week holiday abroad. When I returned he was nowhere to be found. My son John had also been feeding and exercising him. He said Sport had disappeared a few days after I had gone. He was sure he had not left the gates open.

Every effort was made to find him. Advertisements went on radio and in the local paper. I drove the streets for hours, hoping to see him, but in vain. My good friend, Jeff Cocker, came around to offer condolences and brought his pointer with him. The dog roamed around our half-acre and made a point at a thick bush area. When we searched there we found Sport where he had died. I buried him.

CHAPTER 82

The End

My practice was thriving. I employed excellent female staff, some of whom were with me for many years. The nurses were trained to undertake certain jobs and proved to be very efficient in suturing wounds, X-ray techniques, giving hypodermic injections, scaling teeth, changing dressings and assisting with surgical operations. Two of my nurses went to Veterinary College and graduated.

I employed locums to take care of the practice while I made trips to Ireland or Australia. During this time I provided liberally for my family's support. I made no serious attachments for three years then good fortune smiled on me when I met Marilyn who was also separated. We made a good team enjoying the simple things in life, like hiking, boating, Dixieland jazz and being with each other. After uncomplicated divorces we tied the knot with the help of my old friend, Don Pye, who was a marriage commissioner.

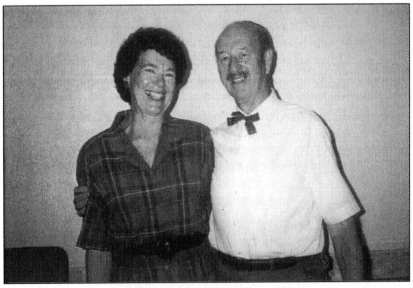

Happily retired with Marilyn, 1989.

The End

The years passed very pleasantly. My children grew up; the two boys are married with young families, the two girls in good positions. When I was just short of age sixty-five I sold my practice and continued the good life with Marilyn.

It was the end of an exciting and rewarding career. There were no great distinctions. I was never involved in professional politics, often being more critical than supportive of the powers that guided our activities.

Like many others of my era we did the best we could at minimal cost. I never charged any member of the cloth for services rendered. Perhaps St. Peter will consider this when the time comes to give an account of myself.